the fast 800
keto

the fast 800 keto

Eat well, burn fat, manage your weight long-term

DR MICHAEL MOSLEY

The content of this book is intended to inform, entertain and provoke your thinking. This is not intended as medical advice. It may, however, make you question current medical and nutritional advice. That is your choice. Neither the author nor the publisher can be held responsible or liable for any loss or claim arising from the use, or misuse, of the content of this book.

Published in 2021 by Short Books,
an imprint of Octopus Publishing Group Ltd
Carmelite House, 50 Victoria Embankment
London, EC4Y 0DZ
www.octopusbooks.co.uk
www.shortbooks.co.uk

An Hachette UK Company
www.hachette.co.uk

10 9 8 7 6 5 4 3 2 1

A CIP catalogue record for this book
is available from the British Library.

ISBN: 978-1-78072-502-4

Cover design by Smith & Gilmour

Recipe consultant: Kathryn Bruton
Recipe editor: Jo Roberts-Miller
Recipe tester: Caroline Barton

Printed and bound in Great Britain by Clays Ltd, Elcograf S.p.A.

This FSC® label means that materials used for the
product have been responsibly sourced

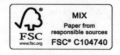

MIX
Paper from
responsible sources
FSC® C104740
FSC
www.fsc.org

CONTENTS

Introduction

In 2012 my world was turned upside down when I was told that a recent blood test had revealed that I had Type 2 diabetes. But threats are sometimes opportunities, so that was also when I decided to re-examine my beliefs and prejudices and find out if there was something I could do to cure myself of what promised to be a nasty, progressive disease.

I did my medical training at the Royal Free Hospital, part of University College, London, in the early 1980s. The Royal Free was a wonderful medical school, but the five years I spent there left me with some pretty fixed beliefs about diet. These included the belief that fats were bad, carbs were good, fasting was ridiculous, probably dangerous, and if you discovered you had Type 2 diabetes then you had better start on medication ASAP, since we all knew that this was a lifelong disease for which there was no cure.

And yet the dean of the Medical School also told us, in a talk he gave on our first day there, that much of what we would learn during our studies would, in time, prove out of date, so we had better keep up with the research. Another thing he said, which I still remember vividly, was that four of us in the room, who had not yet met, would end up marrying each other. He was right. Clare, who is now my wife and who creates all the recipes for our books, was in that room listening to the same talk.

Anyway, fast-forward 30 years and there I was, in early 2012, a happily married father of four (albeit significantly overweight), being told by my lovely GP that I had an incurable disease which I knew would double my risk of heart disease and dementia, take up to 10 years off my life expectancy, probably make me impotent (75% of men with diabetes have erection problems) and increase my risk of having a finger or toe amputated 17-fold. It was a shock. I had already seen the impact that raised blood sugars had had on my father, who had been diagnosed with the same condition in his mid-fifties, at around the age I was then. Despite following medical advice, he had died of diabetes-related complications at the age of 74.

So, rather than follow my own doctor's advice, which was to start on medication, I began to look around for alternatives. And that was when I discovered something called 'intermittent fasting'.

Long story short, I decided to make a film for the eminent BBC Science series, *Horizon*, all about intermittent fasting called 'Eat, Fast, Live Longer'. I wanted to see if I could use this approach to cure myself of Type 2 diabetes, or at least put it into long-term remission, something I was told was impossible.

I went to the US, met a range of experts who were

studying fasting, including Professor Valter Longo, a longevity specialist from the University of Southern California, and Professor Mark Mattson, a leading neuroscientist, based at the National Institute on Aging, and author of dozens of studies on intermittent fasting (or what he more correctly called 'intermittent energy restriction'). Based on his advice, I put myself on a 5:2 intermittent fasting diet, lost 9kg and returned my blood sugars to normal.

That documentary had an astonishing impact. It helped trigger a worldwide interest in different forms of intermittent fasting, ranging from the 5:2 diet to Time-Restricted Eating. It also led me to develop a rapid weight loss programme which forms the basis of this book.

The dean at the Royal Free Medical School was quite right – like so much in medicine, the science behind diets and dieting is constantly evolving as we discover new things about the impact of particular foods on our bodies and brains. And I've made a point of keeping up with the latest research – I really am obsessed with how to improve mood, sleep and metabolic health and finding better ways to lose weight and keep it off.

That's why I've adapted and improved my extremely popular Fast 800 plan to accommodate new findings which highlight the importance of protein in the diet and the many health benefits of combining intermittent fasting with 'going keto'.

Keto – the new/old kid on the block

Like intermittent fasting, keto was barely talked about back in 2012. A standard keto diet is one where you eat large amounts of fat and very little in the way of carbs, normally less than 50g (1.8oz) a day – the amount you'd find in a bagel. The idea is that cutting right back on carbohydrates forces your body to rely on fat as its main source of energy. Without sugar, bread, pasta and rice, your body increasingly depends on your fat stores for fuel, converting them into 'ketone bodies', which put your body into a state of 'ketosis'.

Ketogenic diets promise rapid fat loss and – as a bonus – going keto should stop you from feeling hungry. So it is hardly surprising that keto has taken off, fast. By 2020, 'keto diet' was the most googled diet of all.

When a new diet or health regime suddenly becomes popular, you can be sure it will soon be accompanied by misconceptions and confusion. And I will be honest, when I first heard about the keto diet it struck me as a nutritionist's nightmare. The idea of eating lots of fat and very little in the way of carbs is pretty much the opposite of what most people regard as a healthy, sustainable diet.

Yet I discovered that, at least in the short term, a keto diet can work really well at suppressing appetite and helping people lose weight. It has been used, for more than 100 years, to treat epilepsy (as the brain increasingly relies on ketones for fuel, this reduces brain cell 'excitability' and therefore seizures). And there is mounting evidence that it can help people with Type 2 diabetes return their blood sugars to normal, without medication.

I also discovered that it *is* possible, on a keto diet, to opt for healthy sources of fat, carbs and protein (what I would call a Med-style keto diet), which ensures you get plenty of the right nutrients.

For all these reasons and more, I am now a convert to the keto approach, at least in the short term, which is why it forms the starting point of this new programme.

A combined programme for accelerated weight loss

The Fast 800 Keto is a carefully researched, flexible three-stage programme which starts with a low-calorie ketogenic diet. Most standard keto diets are not calorie restricted, but as I will show you, a short-term low-calorie keto diet, particularly one where you add an element of intermittent fasting, can be very effective for rapid weight loss and restoring health.

When we used this approach for my recent Channel 4 television series 'Lose a Stone in 21 Days', our volunteers were really impressed with how easy they found it. Once they had gone into ketosis they weren't tormented by hunger pangs and they not only lost significant amounts of weight – fast – but also saw big improvements in their blood sugar levels, blood pressure, mood and overall energy.

Stage 1 of the Fast 800 Keto programme involves sticking to around 800–900 calories a day, of which less than 50g come from carbs and at least 50g will come from protein. As I have mentioned, one of the challenges with standard keto, where you are not re-stricting calories, is that you have to eat huge amounts of fat and fatty foods to sustain you. Although that may sound tempting, it is hard to maintain, can soon get very boring and, if you are largely eating meat and dairy (cheese, cream, butter etc), will add significantly to your carbon footprint.

On our healthy, Mediterranean-style keto diet, how-ever, you effectively get the best of both worlds. Al-though fat is an important part of the diet plan, you will be eating healthy fats (olive oil, oily fish, nuts and avocados), and only in calorie-counted moderation. So you do restrict your calories – but not as much as on the Fast 800 (indeed, on days when you are feeling hun-gry, you can choose from a range of keto-friendly 'add-ons' to take your daily quota up to 1000 calories). And yes, you do have to restrict your carbohydrates – but not for long. By Stage 2 of the diet you can start eating more complex carbs, such as lentils or beans, with your fish or omelette (and obviously always lots of greens).

It is also important, during every stage of this diet, to keep eating plenty of protein, well above current rec-ommended levels. Extra protein, combined with some easy-to-do exercises which I describe in Chapter 7, will not only help reduce your appetite and cravings, but ensure that you preserve your muscle mass as you lose weight, fast. You will read far more about the importance of protein, and the major role that lack of good-quality protein has played in our obesity epidemic, in Chapter 2.

If this all sounds a bit technical, you can be reassured that the recipes and menus in the book have been carefully tailored to ensure you hit those calorie, carb and protein targets while also making sure you get all the necessary minerals, vitamins and essential micronutrients. And they are all super easy to follow.

Adrian's story

In 2020 Adrian Vieyra, then aged 44, was one of five people who volunteered to take part in the 'Lose a Stone' TV series. Adrian is married with three children and runs an IT consultancy company. When I met him in June 2020, he described himself as feeling 'old and sluggish'. He said his kids had begun teasing him about the size of his stomach.

I've always been a little bit chubby but I felt that I was good enough. Asian families are feeders, so if you are putting on a bit of weight this is often seen as a healthy thing.

Adrian was determined to tackle his dad bod but didn't know how. He was really worried about getting Covid-19 because he was aware that men of Asian ethnicity who are out of shape are at much higher risk of ending up in intensive care.

When I checked him over, I discovered that he weighed 80.5 kg, and had a Body Mass Index (BMI) of 27.2, which put him in the overweight category. This didn't worry me. What did worry me was that he had a waist size of 42in (107cm), his blood pressure was too high, his blood sugars were borderline prediabetic and his cholesterol was also well above the healthy range. I told him that I could start to transform his health in just three weeks, but he would have to stick closely to the plan.

Being told that I would have to confine myself to 800–900 calories a day was a big shock. I often drink that amount of calories in a night and there you were telling me that this was to be my total calorie allowance for a whole day. I didn't think it was possible in the beginning, to be honest.

It was possible, but it certainly wasn't easy to begin with, as his body started to adapt to the new diet:

I didn't feel good for the first two or three days. I found the cravings hard to deal with and I felt a bit dizzy at times but I did get into a routine – and I love routines. Having the other volunteers do it at the same time was also great; I would've found it harder to do it on my own.

On Day 4, Adrian went into ketosis and suddenly everything became easier.

I felt good. I thought, yes, this is going to work, this is what Michael told me would happen and it has happened.

Apart from the occasional glass of wine, Adrian stuck with the diet and after just three weeks there were some remarkable changes. He lost 6.4kg and 13cm (5in) off his waist. His blood sugars, blood pressure and cholesterol all returned to normal. His blood levels of an enzyme called ALT, which had previously indicated he might have signs of early fatty liver disease, fell by 28%, suggesting his liver had returned to good health.

Adrian moved on to a 3:4 pattern of eating (a form of intermittent fasting where you restrict your calories on four days a week, and eat normally on the other three – more on this later) and lost five more kilos. When we re-tested him six months after starting the diet, he weighed 69kg (he had lost 11kg overall) and, like the others who took part in the Channel 4 programme, showed no signs of the dreaded 'starvation mode' (where, if you don't consume enough calories, your body protects itself by slowing down your metabolism to conserve energy). His metabolic rate was exactly what you would predict for someone his age and weight. He has remained on track ever since.

I learnt so much from you and Clare and I know that this is something I can stick with long term. I keep a fairly close eye on my weight and if it creeps up, I go back to basics and hit it on the head. My

kids are proud of what I've done, and so is my wife.
I can't thank you enough.

What's new?

Since writing *The Fast Diet* in 2012, I have adapted and tweaked the programmes I have presented in response to new research in multiple different ways.

The great thing about this new combined programme is that it not only puts you into ketosis faster than a normal keto diet but is also, I believe, healthier and more sustainable. For this reason, I'm convinced that if you want to improve your health and shift a substantial amount of weight, fast, this is my most effective programme yet.

In this book, after bringing you bang up to date with the latest keto science, exploding myths and showing not only why going Fast Keto is so effective, but crucially how to do it safely, I will take you through a clear, easy-to-follow diet plan, which includes both Clare's delicious recipes and plenty of tips and advice on how to stay on track. People who have done the Fast 800 Keto programme have found, for example, that using 'keto sticks', which tell you when you are in ketosis, is particularly motivating.

Along the way, I am going to introduce you to all sorts of people who have tried this diet, including Dr Gary Lamph, a mental health researcher, who used the Fast 800 Keto approach to shed 4 stone (25kg) in just a few months. As you'll see, this led to big improvements in his physical and mental wellbeing. Drawing on his experience as a cognitive behavioural therapist, helping people overcome their addictions, Gary provides some very valuable advice on how to remain focused and handle any potential weight loss plateau (see Chapter 6).

Gary is just one of many people who have already found this diet life-changing. I hope, if you decide to try it, the same will be true for you.

1

How we got fat

I don't think any of you will be surprised to hear that obesity is a very common problem, worldwide. But it is shocking when you realise just how recently – and how quickly – the world got fat.

Since I was a medical student, 40 years ago, rates of obesity have almost tripled. Two billion adults are now overweight or obese, as are 39 million children under the age of five. If you look at the world's major economies, the US has the highest rates of obesity, closely followed by Mexico, New Zealand, Hungary, Australia and then the UK.[1]

Most of us get fatter as we get older. Between the ages of 20 and 50 we typically put on weight at a rate of about 1lb a year (0.5kg). This doesn't sound that bad, but it means you can find yourself in late middle age 15kg heavier than you were in your twenties.[2]

That's what happened to me. I was under 12 stone (76kg) when I was in my early twenties, and 30 years later I had not only put on about 2½ stone (15kg) but had also developed Type 2 diabetes. Despite the fact that I was snoring the house down and having to buy ever-larger trousers, neither Clare nor I really noticed what was going on. Because it happens so gradually, most people who are overweight or obese, have, like me, little idea how bad things have got. A survey by researchers from University College, London, found that only 11% of women and 7% of men with a BMI over 30 realised that they were obese.[3]

Large waists are now so common we have got used to them. Being a bit on the chubby side is entirely normal. Muffin tops and double chins are everywhere. And, while the fat acceptance movement is right to challenge the stigma around obesity, and celebrating curviness has been, in many ways, a desirable response to unrealistic skinny supermodels, it remains a sad fact that too much fat in the wrong places has serious health consequences.

Which is why, along with the expansion of our waists, there has been a surge in people needing to be treated for weight-related cancers, joint problems, infertility, hypertension and raised blood sugar levels. Around one in three middle-aged people in the UK, US and Australia have metabolic syndrome (a combination of diabetes, raised blood fats, high blood pressure and obesity), which puts them at increased risk of heart disease and stroke. It also increases the risk of dying, prematurely.

Covid has turned this from a distant to a more immediate threat. If you have an underlying health condition, like metabolic syndrome, and contract the virus, then you are also six times more likely to end up in hospital and 12 times more likely to die.[4]

The 'fat makes you fat' fallacy

If you look at graphs showing rates of obesity in the US from 1960 till the present day, you will see a relatively flat line from 1960 to 1975. Then rates start to shoot up, for every age group, from teenagers to 60-year-olds, and every ethnic group.[5]

So what happened? Some blame less exercise, poor sleep or increased anxiety. Others blame the increasing gap between rich and poor. For a long time, it was thought that we were becoming fat because we were eating too much fat; then it was because we were eating too much sugar. I think the evidence points elsewhere. But I will come to that in a moment. Let's first take a quick look at the usual suspects, beginning with fat.

To understand how fat became top villain in the diet wars, we need to go back to 1957, when the American Heart Association went on a mission to persuade the American public to eat less of it. Their real target was saturated fat, which was seen as a major driver of heart disease, but the idea of 'good' fats and 'bad' fats was thought to be too difficult for the public to grasp, so the message was simply 'cut out the fat'. People were encouraged, for example, to cut the fat off meat, eat low-fat dairy products and replace butter with margerine spreads.

The upshot was that, in time, they reduced their intake of beef and full-fat milk, but they didn't pile their shopping trolleys instead with healthy stuff, such as fruit and veg. No, they now ate ever-increasing amounts of heavily marketed, sugary carbohydrates (in the form of low-fat cakes, biscuits, fizzy drinks, etc) and lots of vegetable oils, sales of which soared.

Most of those vegetable oils were highly processed. To turn oil into margarine, the manufacturers used a process called hydrogenation, which in turn led to the production of trans fats. Trans fats, until recently found in most shop-bought biscuits and cakes, are the Lord Voldemort of the fat world. They are major triggers of heart disease. They have been largely phased out.

And further collateral damage was caused by the fact that the 'war on fat' didn't really distinguish between different types of fat. We now know, for example, that the sorts of fat that you find in nuts and oily fish are good for our hearts and our waistlines. Yet to many supporters of the low-fat diet this was heresy.

One of the early and most controversial supporters of the idea that there are 'good fats' and 'bad fats' was Professor Hugh Sinclair, a rather eccentric academic based at the University of Oxford. In the 1940s, Professor Sinclair had travelled to northern Canada to study the Inuit and had become intrigued by their high-fat diet and low rates of heart disease. He wondered whether omega 3 – an essential fatty acid found in oily fish – was protecting the Inuit from heart attacks. In 1956, he wrote a letter to the *Lancet*, entitled 'Deficiency of essential fatty acids and atherosclerosis'. In it he argued, among other things, that heart disease was the result of consuming too little essential fatty acid, rather than too much.

This letter led to such a storm of criticism that for

the next 20 years Sinclair retreated from the medical mainstream. Eventually, in the early 1970s, he decided to test his theory by putting himself on an Inuit diet, eating nothing but seal, oily fish, molluscs and crustaceans. Throughout his experiment, Sinclair measured his bleeding time, the time it took for his blood to clot, by cutting himself every week (he did this because blood clots are one of the key causes of heart attacks and strokes).

While making a series for the BBC on self-experimenters, I decided to repeat his experiment. We tried to import seal from Canada, but it got impounded by customs, so I lived on nothing but fish. Sinclair stuck to his diet for three months; I managed a few weeks.

On his new diet, Sinclair's bleeding time increased from three minutes to a terrifying 50. Mine doubled.

Sinclair had found part of the reason why eating fish oils is so good for the heart: it reduces the tendency of platelets to stick together and thus the risk of forming clots. Since then, many other studies have shown that eating oily fish not only reduces your risk of heart attacks, strokes and death from heart disease, but may also lead to slower rates of mental decline.

Other studies have shown that people who eat fish regularly are much less likely to become depressed and that supplementing your diet with omega 3 can reduce depression.[6] It has also been shown that people who eat oily fish at least once a week have more grey matter in areas like the hippocampus, which is responsible for memory.[7]

Clare and I are big fans of fish, and lots of our recipes are fish based. As well as being rich in omega 3, oily fish is a great source of high-quality protein. Moreover, eating fish has a much lower impact on greenhouse gases than eating meat.[8]

What about cholesterol?

It was not only fat but also cholesterol that took a beating in the 1950s. If it was common sense that eating fat would clog up your arteries, then it was common sense that eating cholesterol would too. After all, it was cholesterol in the arteries that was doing the clogging.

Foods rich in cholesterol, such as eggs, were shunned. Governments warned consumers to eat no more than one egg a week; restaurants pushed the merit of white-only omelettes and supermarkets were stacked to the rafters with foods that declared themselves 'cholesterol-free'.

Yet it turned out that the impact of the cholesterol we eat on the cholesterol levels in our blood is relatively small.

It is a myth that has taken a very long time to die. After years of warning of the dire consequences of eating eggs, the American Heart Association now says, 'In healthy individuals, consumption of an egg a day is acceptable.' In fact, a meta-analysis of studies of more than 200,000 people, followed up for 30 years and published in the *British Medical Journal* in 2020, concluded that 'higher consumption of eggs is not only safe but may actually lower your risk of heart disease'.[9]

The Mediterranean diet

These days fat, at least in part, has been rehabilitated. The Mediterranean diet, widely seen as one of the healthiest diets on the planet, is actually quite high in fat. That's because, as well as plenty of vegetables, fruit and legumes, it contains lots of oily fish, nuts and olive oil.

In a really important study called Predimed, 7447 men and women were randomly allocated to either a standard low-fat diet or a higher-fat Mediterranean diet, in which they ate at least three portions of fruit and vegetables a day, plus fish and legumes (peas, lentils, beans) a minimum of three times a week.[10] They were also encouraged to eat nuts and olive oil and allowed the occasional glass of wine with their meal.

Not surprisingly, people on the Med diet were far more likely to stick to their regime than those on the low-fat diet. Indeed, this trial was stopped early because those on the higher-fat Med diet were doing so much better than those on the low-fat diet, with 30% fewer heart attacks and strokes.

When you look at a breakdown of the macronutrients that people allocated to the Mediterranean diet were eating, it comes in at 41% fat, 41% carbs and 18% protein. It is a diet that is much higher in fat and protein, and lower in carbs, than the sort of diet we are normally recommended.

The rise and fall, rise and fall, then rise again of low-carb diets

Although mainstream medicine has long favoured low-fat diets, for many people it is carbs that are the problem. The thing about carb-rich foods, like biscuits, cake or white rice, is that they are swiftly broken down in your body into sugars, which then cause your blood sugar levels to soar. Your body responds by releasing the hormone insulin, which brings your blood sugars back down again. But a rapid rise and then fall in your blood sugar levels (a blood sugar crash) can make you ravenously hungry. I find that if I have cereal or toast for breakfast, then a couple of hours later I really want to snack. Whereas if I eat something protein-rich, like an omelette, I stay full until much later in the day.

There are good carbs and bad carbs. Many fruits and vegetables are rich in carbs, but they also contain lots of fibre, so your body finds these sorts of food harder to break down. Not surprisingly, you get much smaller blood sugar spikes after eating an apple than after eating an apple pie.

Eating lots of processed carbs, like white rice and packaged bread, is fine if you are doing lots of exercise or hard manual labour, because your muscles will burn through the sugar that is flooding your body. But if you just sit around after a carb-heavy meal, your insulin levels will surge, as your body struggles to bring those blood sugar levels down. And the way insulin does this is by tucking those excess calories away in your fat stores.

Your body has good reasons for doing this – it cannot tolerate high levels of sugar in the blood – but the fact remains, when insulin goes up, fat-burning goes down. And if you have high levels of insulin circulating, it also means there are fewer calories in your bloodstream for the rest of your body to use. So you get hungry and overeat.

Another problem is that our bodies did not evolve to deal with the huge amounts of sugar that we currently consume. So over time, as our levels of body fat rise, we develop something called 'insulin resistance'. Our cells become resistant to the impact of insulin, so our pancreas has to crank out more and more of it to get our blood sugars down. This leads to prediabetes (where your blood sugars are raised, but not yet in the diabetic range), and unless you change your diet and lose weight, it often progresses to Type 2 diabetes and fatty liver disease.

One obvious way to counter this is by eating fewer highly processed carbs.

The first low-carb diet

One of the first people to write about the benefits of going on a low-carb diet (though he didn't call it that), and capture the public imagination, was William Banting, a 19th-century Victorian undertaker who, among other things, prepared elaborate burials for members of the royal family.

Banting's problem was that he was obese; just five and a half feet tall, he weighed over 200lb (90kg). His obesity was so bad that he had to go down the stairs backwards, and on his knees. He had tried everything to lose weight, from Turkish baths to huge amounts of rowing. The trouble was that all the exercise did was make him hungry.

And then, in his early sixties, he went off to visit Dr William Harvey. Dr Harvey told him to cut out sweet, starchy foods, like buttered toast and pastries, and instead stick to meat, fish, vegetables and unsweetened tea. Beer was out, but he was allowed gin, whisky or brandy (all of which are low carb).

Banting stuck to the diet and lost 35lb (17kg) in 36 weeks. He could now walk downstairs, forwards, felt better than he had for years and claimed that his hearing and eyesight had both improved. He wanted to share the good news, so in 1863 he published a pamphlet called 'Letter on Corpulence: Addressed to the Public'.

You can find it online; it is a very short but entertaining read and in many ways it is surprisingly modern. Banting starts by claiming that, 'Of all the parasites that affect humanity, I do not know of, nor can I imagine, any more distressing than that of Obesity', before going on to explain his new diet in a very succinct form:

For breakfast, I take four or five ounces of beef, mutton, kidneys, broiled fish, bacon, or cold meat of any kind except pork; a large cup of tea (without milk or sugar), a little biscuit, or one ounce of dry toast.

For dinner, five or six ounces of any fish except salmon, any meat except pork, any vegetable except potato, one ounce of dry toast, fruit out of a pudding, any kind of poultry or game, and two or three glasses of good claret, sherry, or Madeira – champagne, port and beer forbidden.

For tea, two or three ounces of fruit, a rusk or two, and a cup of tea without milk or sugar.

For supper, three or four ounces of meat or fish, similar to dinner, with a glass or two of claret.

For nightcap, if required, a tumbler of grog – (gin, whiskey, or brandy, without sugar) – or a glass or two of claret or sherry.

And that was it as far as Banting's dieting advice went. But his pamphlet struck a chord; it sold like crazy, and the first low-carb diet was born. Banting himself lived to the ripe old age of 82; he died of pneumonia.

The Atkins diet

After Banting's death, interest in his diet faded away and it would be a hundred years before another low-carb diet book caught the public imagination in such a vivid fashion. This time it was *Dr Atkins' Diet Revolution*, which was published in 1972. Written by a former cardiologist, Robert Atkins, who had lost lots of weight by going low carb, it became one of the bestselling books of all time.

Doctors hated the Atkins diet, which focused on eating foods like cream, cheese, bacon and red meat, while avoiding potatoes, rice and wholegrains. But most people who tried it lost weight without having to worry about calories, which is why it became insanely popular.

The Atkins empire rose to giddy heights (at one point 10% of Americans were said to be on the Atkins diet) … and then it all fell apart. In 2003, Robert Atkins died, after slipping on ice and hitting his head. Although his widow refused to allow an autopsy, his medical records were leaked. These revealed that at his time of death he was hugely overweight and had signs of advanced heart disease. In 2005, the company he had founded, Atkins Nutritionals, filed for bankruptcy.

But the low-carb diet didn't die, and many doctors, particularly those who see and treat patients with Type 2 diabetes, became interested. One of them is a GP, called Dr David Unwin, whom I know very well.

Dr Unwin's breakthrough trial

As a GP, David had, for most of his life, given his patients the conventional low-fat advice. But he had become gloomy about its impact. He told me that between 1986 and 2012, there was an eightfold increase in the number of patients in his practice with Type 2 diabetes, many of them shockingly young.

Then, in 2012, a former diabetes patient turned up – 10% lighter and free of diabetes. 'She mystified me. But I am always fascinated by stories of success so I asked her what she had done.'

She replied, 'You're not going to like this, doctor.' She had read about the benefits of a low-carb, high-fat diet and given it a go.

David did some research and decided to do a small trial. He recruited 19 patients who had Type 2 diabetes or prediabetes and gave them a very simple diet sheet.

'Reduce starchy carbohydrates a lot (remember they are just concentrated sugar),' it read. 'If possible, cut out the white stuff like bread, pasta, rice. As for sugar – cut it out altogether, although it will be in the blueberries, strawberries and raspberries you are allowed to eat free-ly.'

Instead, patients were encouraged to eat more protein, butter, full-fat yoghurt and olive oil: 'Eating lots of veg with protein and fats leaves you properly full in a way that lasts,' he wrote in capital letters.

The patients who took part in this early trial started out with an average weight of 100kg (220lb) and over the eight months of the trial lost over 9kg (20lb), much of it around the waist.

By the end, only two of the 19 still had raised blood sugars and even they had seen a huge improvement. There were also big improvements in blood pressure and cholesterol levels, despite the fact that his patients were now eating far more eggs and butter.

Since then, David, who is an expert clinical adviser for the Royal College of GPs, has helped more than 100 patients with Type 2 diabetes come off drugs and published more studies. He, and other GPs like him, have not only changed their patients, but also changed how doctors view low-carb diets, particularly in the context of Type 2.

Ultra-processed foods – the real villain

Although I believe that lower-carb diets can be very helpful, particularly for people with Type 2 diabetes, I don't think that most people get fat simply because they are eating a lot of rice and potatoes. It is also hard to blame sugar for the present obesity crisis, as consumption of sugar has been falling in most developed countries over the last decade, while rates of obesity have been rising. And as I regularly point out to people who claim that sugar is addictive, I feel no compulsion to eat sugar cubes or dip a spoon into a bowl of sugar and snack on that. Nor, I suspect, do most people.

No, I think the real villain, the main driver of obesity worldwide, is the rise and rise of ultra-processed food, the sort of brightly packaged, aggressively marketed products that fill our supermarket shelves. Typically, they are high in both fat and sugar, along with mysterious preservatives and emulsifiers (E numbers). I suspect the main reason that David's patients are losing weight and getting healthier is not just that they are cutting down on the carbs, but that they are eliminating the ultra-processed foods. We are going to take a closer look at the science behind this claim in the next few pages.

What is an ultra-processed food?

In 2009, a team led by Carlos Monteiro, Professor of Nutrition and Public Health at the University of Sao Paulo in Brazil, published a hugely important paper called 'The issue is not food, nor nutrients, so much as processing'.[11]

They argued that while people have, for decades, been blaming fats and carbs for the rise in obesity, they have largely ignored the importance of processing, the extent to which the foods we eat have been manipulated and altered by the big food manufacturers before they reach our plates.

So, they set about identifying different categories of food, ranging from those that have been minimally processed to those that are ultra-processed, and created the NOVA classification system.[12]

NOVA breaks down foods into the following groups:

Unprocessed or minimally processed foods

These are foods that are fresh, frozen, pasteurised, fermented, bottled or packaged. They are not all completely untouched, as nature intended them, but whatever processing they have been through is minimal. The important thing is that there are no added sugars, oils or fats.

Foods that fall into this category include: fruit, vegetables, rice, legumes (i.e. lentils, chickpeas), meat, poultry, fish and seafood (fresh or frozen). Then there are eggs, oats, pasta, couscous and polenta. Nuts, without added salt, are also part of this group, as are herbs and spices, milk and plain yoghurt, tea, coffee and water.

Processed foods

These are often foods taken from the first group, with a bit of salt or sugar added. They include fresh bread, salted, cured or smoked meats, tinned fish, tinned fruit, butter, cheese, wine and beer.

Ultra-processed foods

The foods in this group are not so much foods as formulations: they are made in factories and are designed to imitate the taste and smell of fresh or minimally processed foods, while actually being produced out of cheap industrial ingredients and additives. They contain lots of sugars, fats and salt, as well as, according to the *World Nutrition Journal* in 2016, 'dyes and other colours, colour stabilisers, flavours, flavour enhancers, non-sugar sweeteners, and processing aids such as carbonating, firming, bulking and anti-bulking, de-foaming, anti-caking and glazing agents, emulsifiers, sequestrants and humectants'. The reason manufacturers add these strange-sounding ingredients to their products is to give them a long shelf life and to make them 'hyperpalatable'. In other words, to keep us coming back for more. The ultimate aim of the Big Food manufacturers is, of course, to make Big Bucks. And they certainly do.

The foods in the group include some pretty obvious candidates, like chicken nuggets, burgers, chips, pizzas, hotdogs, pre-packaged meals, fizzy drinks and packaged fruit juices. But it also includes most mass-produced breads (brown as well as white, just look at what it says on the label), shop-bought biscuits, cakes, buns and sweetened breakfast cereals.

Mass-produced ice-cream, fruit yoghurts, chocolate, sweets, crisps, energy bars, margarine and pretty well anything that says 'instant'– i.e. instant noodles, soups, desserts – also fall into this category.

Vegans and vegetarians are being increasingly targeted with ultra-processed convenience foods, such as vegan sausage rolls. Just because it's plant based doesn't mean it's healthy.

How can you spot an ultra-processed food? Read the label. If there are five or more ingredients, and those ingredients include numbers or have names you don't recognise, the chances are it's ultra-processed.

Sue's story

Sue Bernard, a former IT manager, knows exactly what it is like to be in thrall to ultra-processed food. In her case, the problem was late-night grazing.

I would have a healthy dinner, and then after dinner I was dreadful. I ate crisps and chocolate and ice cream. It was non-stop. It was a complete compulsion. And I would even say to my husband, 'Why am I doing this? Why am I going back into the kitchen to open the fridge and eat more chocolate when I know I cannot be hungry?' It was almost as if I had a fat wish; we talk about a death wish but this was definitely a fat wish. It was as if I wasn't in control.

I was stick thin as a child. We didn't have a car, I walked everywhere. Until my first son was born, I was nine stone and a size 10. Then I had three children and with each child I put on a bit of weight and didn't lose it. Over the years I've tried different ways to lose weight but none of them worked. The catalyst moment was when I saw a photo of myself and I thought I can't share that – I look huge. I remember the moment incredibly clearly – it was the 10th December 2020.

At that point, Sue was 14½ stone (92kg). She had arthritis in her knees and constant back pain:

All the problems you have when you are hugely overweight. And I kept thinking, I'm not going to live to see my family growing up.

She saw my Channel 4 documentary, 'Lose a Stone in 21 days', and decided to put herself on my diet.

I saw those people lose all that weight and I thought, 'I can do that'. I decided this would be the start of a new life. It was as if a switch went in my head.

To start with it wasn't easy:

A couple of nights in the first week I wanted desperately to eat chocolate or ice cream so I went to bed. I started drinking lots of water. In the morning I started drinking black coffee instead of white coffee so I could still enjoy my coffee.

I lost 35lb (16kg) in the first 12 weeks and then I switched on to the 5:2 diet. I have now lost 60lb (27kg). I went from a size 20 to a size 12. Though to be honest it's not really about being size 12, but I know that being size 12 means that I'm healthy.

Now I've lost the weight I can bend my knees, something that I couldn't do before.

We have a couple of small dogs and I do take them out for a walk every day, a couple of miles. When I realised I could move more I joined a local gym and three or four mornings a week I go to the gym and do the bike and the rowing machine. I do crunches and stretches.

How do I keep on course? I always plan. It is a way of life and not just a way of eating. I don't want the sweet things any more, I don't crave them.

My youngest son said to me the other day, 'Do you know what, Mum, I thought you were on your way to an early grave and now you have a real brightness, a real spring in your step.' I thought that was lovely.

Big Food

It might shock you to find out (it certainly shocked me) that just 10 companies control most of the world's large food and drink brands. Some of them are names you will know; some are less familiar. The Big 10 are: Nestlé, PepsiCo, Coca-Cola, Unilever, Danone, General Mills, Kellogg's, Mars, Associated British Foods and Mondelez.

The biggest of the big beasts are Nestlé, Coca-Cola and PepsiCo. They each own dozens of other brands, and are worth, together, more than $700 billion. If you had invested in them when Covid struck in March 2020, you would have made a killing because sales of their incredibly profitable products soared during lockdown.

Along with additives and strange-sounding chemicals, ultra-processed foods tend to come wrapped in lots of packaging.

In 2020, Nestlé, PepsiCo and Coca-Cola were rated, by the pressure group 'Break Free from Plastic' as 'the top plastic polluters' for the third year in a row. This claim was based on a survey they carried out of 55 countries, which showed that the packaging and containers produced by the Big Three were the ones the group's volunteers were most likely to find discarded on beaches, and in rivers and parks.[13] They are certainly the most common forms of litter I find on the road outside my house, along with cigarette packets and energy drink bottles.

I suppose this is not surprising, because, according to a report by the Ellen MacArthur Foundation, these three companies produce over 6.7 million tonnes of plastic every year and recycle less than 10% of it.[14]

How can you cut back on ultra-processed foods? The advice of the Brazilian scientists who are behind the NOVA classification is, as you might expect, to go for water and milk instead of soft drinks, fruit and nuts instead of cakes and biscuits, and to cook at home rather than rely on takeaways, pre-prepared frozen meals and shop-bought desserts.

The impact of ultra-processed foods on our health

There have been a number of studies which suggest that eating more ultra-processed food increases your risk of hypertension, heart disease, Type 2 diabetes and some cancers.[15]

Most recently, in an influential Spanish study, published in 2019, 19,899 Spanish university graduates, with an average age of 38 years, were asked to complete a detailed dietary questionnaire and then followed for an average of 10 years.[16]

The researchers found that people eating lots of ultra-processed foods (more than four servings per day) were 62% more likely to have died during that time, from all causes, compared with those eating fewer than two servings a day. It was a clear dose response; in other words, for each additional daily serving of ultra-processed food, your chance of dying over the following 10 years increased by 18%.

The link between consumption of these foods and poor health, not only physical but also mental – as evidenced by the higher rates of depression and anxiety – is very clear. But to what extent can we blame ultra-processed foods for the expansion of our waistlines? And what is it about these foods that means we find them so hard to resist?

The rise in obesity, worldwide, which began in the 1980s, certainly coincided with an increase in marketing and consumption of ultra-processed foods. When I was in medical school, back in the 1980s, the average UK family diet was made up of roughly 58% fresh ingredients and 26% convenience foods.

By 2014 those numbers had reversed, with us Brits getting 57% of our calories from ultra-processed food, which also accounted for two thirds of the sugar we were eating. And the trend has continued. Countries which have some of the highest rates of obesity in the world, like the US, UK and Australia, are also countries where many people are getting well over half their calories from ultra-processed food.

When you look at the people in those countries who are eating the most ultra-processed food, they are also the ones who have the highest rates of obesity and all the complications that come with being obese, such as Type 2 diabetes.

And what is really concerning, for the future, is that it is the young who are consuming ultra-processed foods in the largest amounts. A recent study from the US showed that over the last 20 years, the percentage of calories that children and adolescents get from ultra-processed foods jumped from 61% to 67%.[17] Since we know that eating ultra-processed foods not only makes you fat but also contributes to anxiety and depression, this is a very worrying trend.

My big fat ultra-processed diet experiment

In 2020, I decided to do a self-experiment in which I would put myself on a medium-level ultra-processed food diet for an Australian documentary called 'Australia's Health Revolution'. I didn't go crazy; I just moved onto a fairly typical Australian diet in which at least half my calories came from ultra-processed food.

I went back to eating cereal for breakfast, fruit yoghurts, plenty of snacks and some microwaveable frozen meals. Several times a week I also went to a fast-food restaurant and had a burger and chips, with Coke to wash it down, or fried chicken and chips, again with a sweet, fizzy drink.

I had my weight, waist, blood sugars and blood pressure measured before starting on this diet, and then at the end of two weeks.

At the start I quite enjoyed it, eating the sort of food I hadn't had for a long time. I also ate foods I had never tried before, like the cheese sausage, a sausage stuffed with cheese which I am told is particularly popular with Australian truckers. When I checked out the ingredients of a typical cheese sausage online, this is what I saw:

Pork, water, cheese, milk, potato starch, sodium nitrite (a preservative), dextrose (a form of sugar), diphosphate, sodium acetate, sodium carbonate and sodium ascorbate.

Yummy. One of the things I quickly noticed, on my new diet, was that within hours of eating, I would get really hungry and crave more junk food. I soon started sleeping badly, snoring loudly, and in a matter of days I felt far more lethargic than normal. I was tracking my blood sugar levels throughout the two weeks and within a few days they started to rise, alarmingly. I was more anxious than normal, and that contributed to my need for more comfort food.

After two weeks, I did repeat tests. By now I had put on 3kg, my waist had expanded by around 3cm and my blood sugar levels had gone into the diabetic range.

My blood pressure had also soared to 140/90, which alarmed the GP who tested me.

So I got out my keto urine sticks (in order to be able to measure levels of ketones in my urine) and put myself on the Fast 800 Keto diet. Within 10 days I had shed the weight and when I was retested, everything had returned to normal, which was a huge relief.

A friend of mine, Dr Chris van Tulleken, who is particularly worried about the impact that ultra-processed foods are having on the bodies and brains of children (as I pointed out earlier, they eat far more of the stuff than adults), did a similar self-experiment for the BBC for a programme called 'What Are We Feeding our Kids?'.

He went further than I did. For a month, 80% of everything he ate came in the form of ultra-processed food, such as cocoa-flavoured breakfast cereals, chicken nuggets and microwaveable lasagnes. Eighty per cent sounds like a lot, but that is what around one in five Brits eat.

Like me, he soon started piling on the weight. He slept badly, felt sluggish and became constipated. He also started craving more and more junk food.

In four weeks, he put on 6.5kg (over a stone), much of it fat, and there was a significant rise in his appetite hormones. But the most striking changes took place in his brain. He had his brain scanned before and after the experiment, and to his horror discovered that eating all that ultra-processed food had, in a month, literally re-wired his brain.

Rachel Batterham, who is Professor of Obesity,

Diabetes and Endocrinology at University College, London, and who supervised his self-experiment, told Chris that she had detected a lot of new connections in his brain, many of them between the reward centres and the cerebellum, an area that controls automatic behaviours. In other words, he appeared to have been reprogrammed by his new diet to seek out and eat even more of these unhealthy foods. Chris managed to lose the weight he had put on, but who knows if his brain will ever fully recover.

The sceptical researcher

Further direct evidence that ultra-processed foods are behind the rise in obesity comes from an experiment carried out by Dr Kevin Hall, an American researcher who started out as a sceptic. He thought it was very unlikely that ultra-processed foods were as bad as people were claiming, so he decided to do an experiment to find out.[18]

In 2018, he and his team recruited 20 healthy volunteers, 10 men and 10 women, and asked them to spend four weeks at the National Institutes of Health Clinical Center, near Washington DC, where they could be closely monitored. They were randomly allocated to two weeks of eating meals that were made up of either ultra-processed foods or minimally processed foods. Then they swapped over for two weeks.

To give you some idea of what they were fed, an

ultra-processed breakfast might consist of a bagel with cream cheese and bacon, while the unprocessed breakfast was porridge with bananas, walnuts and milk.

The clever thing was that the ultra-processed meals and the minimally processed meals all contained exactly the same balance of calories, sugars, fibre, fat and carbohydrates. The volunteers were told they could eat as much or as little as they wanted of each meal and of various snacks, which were readily available.

So what happened? Well, although the volunteers said that they found the meals, ultra-processed or not, equally tasty and filling, it turned out that which regime they were on had a big impact on how much and how quickly they ate.

When the volunteers were eating the ultra-processed food, they consumed about 500 calories more per day than they did on the unprocessed diet. Yes, an extra 500 calories. As a result, they put on an average of 0.9kg, or 2lb, over the two weeks that they were on the ultra-processed diet, and lost roughly the same amount while they were on the unprocessed diet.

Why did this happen? Dr Hall is not entirely sure. The volunteers ate the ultra-processed food faster, probably because it was generally softer and easier to swallow. And the faster you eat, the more you eat.

One way to reduce the amount you eat, of course, is to linger over your meal, and give yourself time to realise that you are feeling satisfied. Even more important, though, is to ensure that you are eating foods packed with fibre.

Foods that are high in fibre, such as veggies, legumes, fruit and wholegrains, not only provide volume and stop you getting constipated, but also delay stomach emptying and slow down the passage of food through your intestines, which means that you feel full for longer on fewer calories. Furthermore, fibre feeds the good bacteria that live in your gut – your microbiome – which help keep your brain and immune system in good shape. The problem with many convenience foods is that – in order to make them palatable and give them that long shelf life – they have had most of their fibre removed.

Another possible explanation for why people ate more on the ultra-processed food diet – which Dr Hall plans to test in future experiments – is that, although the meals were matched for carbs and fat, they were not precisely matched for protein. Fourteen per cent of the calories in the ultra-processed foods were made up of protein, versus 15.6% of the calories in the healthier meals. The difference appears small, but Dr Hall thinks it may, nonetheless, have contributed to the very different outcomes.

Summary

- Although fats, carbs and sugar have in turn been blamed for the current obesity crisis, there is mounting evidence that the real problem is ultra-processed food, which is typically high in poor-quality fat, carbs, sugar and salt, making it incredibly calorific and hard to resist. And as Dr Chris van Tulleken discovered, once you start eating these foods they can mess with your brain.

- We know that eating lots of ultra-processed foods, particularly when you are young, contributes to anxiety and depression.

- Not only are ultra-processed foods full of the unhealthy stuff, they also tend to be low in fibre, so we go on eating them without feeling sated. On top of that, given that eating fibre is essential for keeping your gut bacteria in good shape, a diet high in ultra-processed foods is going to damage your microbiome and lead to inflammation in the gut.

- And finally, ultra-processed foods tend to be low in protein, and as we are about to discover, protein is a key driver of appetite.

2

Why we need to eat more protein

The three main macronutrients that our bodies need are protein, fats and carbohydrates. These are our 'macros'. We need micronutrients such as vitamins and minerals too, of course, but most of us get what we need from our usual diet.

The traditional dietary advice has been to pile our plates with plenty of carbs, like bread, pasta, rice and potatoes, because they provide energy, while low-carbers and classic keto dieters emphasise the importance of eating lots and lots of fat (oil, butter, cream, etc). But I am fascinated by emerging science which shows the vital importance of that other macronutrient, protein (eggs, fish, meat, tofu, and so on) – and mounting evidence that, far from eating too much of it, as many dietitians claim, many of us aren't eating enough.

We know that fat is vital as an energy reserve, for insulation and protection of our organs, and for absorption and transport of fat-soluble vitamins. Carbs provide energy for our muscles and central nervous system during movement and exercise. Carbs, in the form of grains, fruit and veg, are also our main source of fibre. But protein is, in many ways, even more essential. We need it to build muscles, enzymes and much of the infrastructure of our bodies. Every cell in our body contains protein, and eating enough of it is absolutely vital for growth and repair.

Protein is made up of strings of different amino acids. Our body needs 20 amino acids in all, and can make 11 of them on its own. However, there are nine 'essential amino acids', so called because our body cannot make them. We have to get them from the food we eat.

Foods such as meat, fish, eggs and dairy contain high levels of all nine essential amino acids. It can be difficult to get enough if you are on a vegetarian or vegan diet because plant-based foods not only tend to be lower in protein, they are also 'incomplete' – i.e. they contain lower levels of at least one essential amino acid. The secret is to mix and match.

Ultra-processed foods, particularly snacks, normally contain little quality protein – partly because protein is expensive, at least compared to fats and carbs. Instead, the manufacturers use artificial flavourings to try to fool our taste buds into thinking we are eating protein, when we're not.

Beef-flavoured crisps, for example, taste as if they contain lots of protein, but actually consist mainly of carbs and fat. There is just 1.6g of protein in a smallish bag, so if you ate nothing but crisps you would need to eat at least 30 bags to meet the current recommended protein requirements, which is 50g a day, and to achieve that you would be consuming 4000 calories a day, along with three times your daily salt allowance.

Two leading Australian researchers have developed a theory called the 'Protein Leverage Hypothesis', which argues that we have a specific appetite for protein and that the relatively low levels of protein in ultra-processed foods have been one of the major drivers behind the current obesity epidemic. This theory is currently gathering a lot of fans (including me).

The Protein Leverage Hypothesis

Professor David Raubenheimer and Professor Steve Simpson both work for the Charles Perkins Centre, at the University of Sydney, where Steve is also the academic director. It is a very unusual place, where they bring researchers from all sorts of different areas of science together with the goal of improving global health by finding new ways to combat chronic lifestyle diseases.

They have recently written a brilliant book called *5 Appetites* (also called *Eat Like the Animals* in Australia and the USA), which distils a lot of their research. In the book, they claim that we don't have just one appetite, for food in general, we actually have five: one each for protein, fat, carbs, calcium and salt. We have sensors in our mouth, in the lining of our gut and within our brain which detect the presence of these nutrients. If we don't get enough of any of them, we develop cravings.

But it is the need for protein that dominates the

others. Or, as they put it, 'We overeat fats and carbs not because the appetites for these nutrients are stronger, but because the appetite for protein is strongest of all! If protein is diluted in the food supply, we overeat until we satisfy our protein appetite. On high-protein diets, the protein appetite will be satisfied sooner – when fewer total calories have been eaten. This is what we call the Protein Leverage Effect.'[19]

In other words, if we are surrounded by foods which are rich in fats and carbs, but low in protein, we go on eating and eating with no restraint until we have satisfied our protein hunger.

That's why it's so easy for some of us to polish off a big bag of crisps or a packet of biscuits in one sitting. A chocolate biscuit, of the type I love, is 60% carbs and only 6% protein. If I ate all the biscuits in a packet (which I am quite capable of doing), I would consume 1300 calories (almost my daily allowance), but only 16g of protein. No wonder I can just keep going.

If, on the other hand, I was offered a plate of fish or chicken, which comes in at close to 30% protein, I wouldn't be able to eat anything like as much, calorie wise. My protein appetite would soon be satisfied.

The perfect swarm

I first met Steve through a mutual friend, back in 2015. Born in Australia, Steve studied at the University of Queensland, did his PhD at King's College London on 'locust feeding physiology' and then spent 22 years at my old university, Oxford, before returning to Australia to become director of the Charles Perkins Institute.

It was that early research for his PhD that led him to concentrate on locusts when he and David started to study the impact of protein on human hunger signals. One of the key things they showed early on was that they could make locusts extremely fat or very thin, simply by altering the protein content of their food. If you give locusts a low-protein diet, they will eat and eat, until they become fat, in a desperate attempt to top up their protein levels. Steve told me that, among other things, this drive for protein helps explain why locusts swarm.

Locusts are normally solitary creatures, but every so often they get together in giant swarms, which devastate the countryside. These swarms are so dramatic that they are mentioned in the Quran and the Bible. Three thousand years ago, the Chinese created the role of 'anti-locust operative' to try to manage them.

The key trigger for the swarms, as Steve explained, is a shortage of protein in the plants that the locusts normally feed on, which means they have to go looking for other sources of protein-rich foods. And for most locusts, the closest and most convenient source of a protein snack is another locust. So they become cannibalistic. What you are really seeing in a swarm are locusts trying to eat the locusts in front of them and avoid being eaten by the ones behind.

Fortunately, we do not usually turn cannibal when we are running low on protein, but a shortage can drive us to overeat. Steve and David demonstrated this in an elegant experiment they published in 2011 called 'Testing protein leverage in lean humans: a randomised controlled experimental study'.[20]

For this experiment, they recruited 22 healthy volunteers and kept them locked away in hotel-style accommodation in Sydney University. They were allowed out for supervised walks, but the researchers kept a very close eye on them to check they weren't sneaking in any extra food.

On three separate occasions, the volunteers took part in four-day experiments, during which meals were provided, as well as access to lots of different snacks. The volunteers didn't know the real purpose of the experiment and they weren't told that their meals, although matched for calories, contained very different levels of protein.

On one of their four-day visits, the meals contained 10% protein, on the next it was 15% and on the third it was 25%. What the scientists wanted to see was whether this would make any difference to how much the volunteers ate, and if so, how much. It certainly had an effect. Without realising it, the volunteers ate, on average, 210 calories more per day when they were on the low-protein diet than they did on the higher-protein diet.

Do that on a regular basis and you would soon find yourself piling on the weight.

The volunteers also reported feeling much hungrier

a couple of hours after eating the low-protein breakfast, despite eating the same number of calories as on higher-protein days. That is certainly what I find. When I eat eggs or fish for breakfast, I stay full until lunchtime. If I eat the same number of calories in the form of cereal or toast, I am craving a snack by mid-morning.

What I found particularly interesting in this experiment was that most of the extra calories the volunteers ate came from eating savoury snacks, not from eating bigger meals or the sugary snacks that were also freely available.

So are we eating less protein than we used to?

A key claim of the Protein Leverage Hypothesis is that to satisfy our protein hunger, most of us need to get around 15–20% of our calories in the form of protein. As their Sydney experiment showed, go below 15% and your protein hunger will make you want to eat more.

So does this help explain our obesity epidemic? They think it does. Far from eating too much protein, as many claim, an analysis of data collected by the US Department of Agriculture between 1970 and 2010 reveals that the proportion of protein in the American diet fell, while consumption of fat and carbs soared. And over those 40 years, rates of obesity tripled.[21]

According to a Pew Research study published in

2016,[22] between 1970 and 2010:

- The average American increased the number of calories they consumed by around 500 a day, up from an average of 2000 to 2500. A lot of these extra calories were in the form of snacks.

- Consumption of meat and fish remained stable, but there were big falls in consumption of protein-rich eggs and milk.

- By 2010, Americans were eating more than three times as much vegetable oil – mainly in the form of highly processed soybean, corn or rapeseed – as they were in 1970.

- They were eating less cane sugar, but far more corn-derived sweeteners, such as high-fructose corn syrup.

- And they were eating far more bread, pastries and other baked goods – roughly 122lb per person per year.

The increase in the consumption of vegetable oil is because people are eating so much more junk food, which is often fried in it, while the heavy marketing of ultra-processed foods has led to a huge increase in easily digestible carbs, like breakfast cereals.

Tragically, people with metabolic diseases, like Type 2 diabetes, are still being told to eat a low-protein, high-carbohydrate diet, which puts them at much greater risk of obesity and ill-health.

A recent study by researchers at Ohio State University,

which looked at the dietary habits of a representative sample of more than 23,000 Americans with Type 2 diabetes, found that more than half were eating less than the recommended daily intake of protein (which is a miserly 50g a day). Instead, they were filling up on sugars and unhealthy carbs.[23]

Their low-protein diet had a big impact on their strength and ability to do even basic tasks like 'stooping, crouching, kneeling, standing for long periods, and pushing or pulling large objects'.

What level of protein should we aim for?

Current guidelines say women should be aiming to eat around 45g of protein a day, and men should be aiming for 55g. But many experts think these numbers are far too low. If you follow these guidelines, and also stick to the recommended daily calorie intake (2000 calories a day for women, 2500 for men), then you will only be getting 9% of your diet in the form of protein.

This is how you do that calculation:

There are 4 calories in a gram of protein. So a woman eating 45g of protein would be consuming 180 calories a day in protein. Which is 180/2000 x 100 = 9% of her recommended daily calorie allowance.

For a man, 55g of protein means 220 calories, which is 220/2500 x 100 = 8.8%.

A classic Mediterranean diet, of the sort used in the Predimed study, contains around 18% protein, which is nearly twice the recommended level and gets you much closer to the Protein Leverage Effect ideal. As you get older it becomes even more important to raise your protein intake to avoid age-related muscle loss. A recent review of the evidence concluded that 'higher intakes of high-quality protein (1.0–1.5g/kg of body weight per day), evenly distributed throughout the day, may maximally stimulate muscle protein synthesis, thereby contributing to maintaining muscle mass in older adults'.[24]

What this means is that someone who weighs 80kg, as I do, should be aiming for at least 80–120g of protein a day, which is far higher than the current official recommended levels.

Protein doesn't just help strengthen and build muscles – it keeps your bones healthy too. According to the International Osteoporosis Foundation, eating more protein (a lot more) 'is associated with higher bone density, a slower rate of bone loss, and reduced risk of hip fracture, provided that dietary calcium intakes are adequate'. In other words, if you want to keep your bones strong as you get older, you had better increase the protein (and calcium) in your diet.[25]

Why should you need more protein as you get older? Well, it is mainly because our ageing bodies are not as good at absorbing or making use of protein as they used to be. And too little protein not only leads to muscle shrinkage but also puts you at increased risk of infection and frailness. This seems to be especially true in women.

In the Framingham Heart Study Offspring, in which 2917 middle-aged men and women were followed for an average of 23 years, they found that women who were eating at least 90g of protein a day scored better on measures of frailty, including things like grip strength, being able to go up and down stairs, walk half a mile or dress themselves, than women who were eating 60g of protein a day, or less.[26]

It is also particularly important that pregnant women get enough protein. In a study carried out at the John Hunter Hospital, in Newcastle, Australia, 179 women were asked to fill in detailed food questionnaires during their pregnancy.[27] They also had detailed ultra-sound scans done at four different points during their pregnancy, so researchers could see how their babies were growing.

What the researchers found is that the mothers who were eating relatively low levels of protein (less than 16% of their daily diet) had babies with high levels of fat around the tummy, which is unhealthy. Having a chubby baby is fine, but you want them to have fat around the thighs and arms, not the tummy.

For these reasons, another recent review recommended that pregnant women should be eating 1.2–1.5g/kg per day of protein, which is, again, well above current recommended levels.

KayleighAnn – the junk-food vegan

Lots of people go vegan for ethical and health reasons, but just because your diet is vegan it doesn't mean it is necessarily healthy. When I met 29-year-old KayleighAnn, she told me that her friends called her a 'junk-food vegan'. She weighed over 17 stone (108kg), was anaemic and had the fitness level of someone twice her actual age. Although she was on a plant-based diet, a lot of the foods she was eating were ultra-processed, high in fat and carbs, but low in protein. In fact, a food diary, which I asked her to keep, revealed that she was only eating around 30g of protein a day.

So, I recommended she up the protein in her diet, by including more chickpeas, tempeh, quinoa and edamame beans. I also got her to cut down on the junk food and become more active (see Chapter 7).

By making these relatively simple changes, she lost nearly a stone (6kg) in three weeks and recently ran a half marathon.

Can you overdo protein consumption?

You might be thinking that when it comes to protein, more is always better. But that isn't necessarily true. According to Professor Simpson, their experiments, and those of many others since, have shown that animals that are put on a very high-protein, low-carb diet tend to die younger. That's because, at least in mice and other experimental-study animals, a high-protein, low-carb diet seems to supercharge the metabolic pathways that lead to rapid ageing, switching off repair mechanisms and promoting changes that can lead to cancer and heart disease.

A very high-protein diet might help keep you slim, but it won't necessarily be healthier for you in the long term. There are also concerns that eating lots of protein could be bad for your kidneys, so if you have kidney disease you need to be especially wary of going on a very high-protein diet.

That said, in the short term, a diet comprising anything up to 30% protein seems to be safe – although most long-term studies suggest we should be aiming to eat 15–20%, with the amount you eat going up after the age of 65, when, as I just pointed out, you need to eat more protein to preserve your muscle mass.[28]

When you start on the Fast 800 Keto diet (Stage 1) you will be getting 20–25% of your diet as high-quality protein (around 50g a day). Combined with the fact that you are in ketosis, this should help suppress your appetite.

When you move on to Stage 2, you will be eating more calories, so we also recommend you boost the amount of protein you are eating, to ensure it remains at around 20% of your total calories. This should take you up to 60–70g a day.

By the time you reach Stage 3 – a Mediterranean-style diet – the amount of protein in your diet still needs to be 15–20% of your total calories, which for most women means eating 70–80g of protein a day, and for men 90–100g. As I mentioned earlier, this is *nearly twice the amount that is routinely recommended.*

But remember, if you have a kidney problem, there is a risk that a higher protein diet could make it worse, so do talk to your doctor.

Summary

- Eating adequate amounts of good-quality protein is vital for keeping you strong and slim. This is particularly important as you get older, or if you work out a lot.

- We have a powerful appetite for protein, and if you aren't getting enough, or if it is being 'diluted' by lots of fat and carbs (so that the percentage of protein in your diet dips below 15%), you will find that you are often hungry.

- One of the tricks that the producers of ultra-processed foods play on us is adding flavours that fool our taste buds into thinking they are eating something that is protein-rich, when it is not. That is one of the reasons why we go on eating more and more of these foods, in a desperate search for protein that is not there.

Good sources of protein

Meat is a particularly rich source, delivering 33g of protein for every 100g of meat (a small serving).

Fish is also rich in protein, with 21g per 100g. It doesn't have to be fresh - it can be frozen or canned. Oily fish is also a great source of omega 3 fatty acids (good for the heart and the brain).

Greek yoghurt. I love it with some berries as a quick breakfast or dessert. It typically contains twice the amount of protein as other yoghurts, with a 200g serving providing around 17g.

Nuts. A small handful (something like nine almonds) can make a filling snack. They contain lots of fibre and a couple of grams of protein as well.

Eggs. I love eggs. They make a great breakfast and each one delivers around 7g of protein.

Lentils. I used to hate them but they have become one of my favourite foods. One cup of cooked lentils (200g) provides 21g of protein.

Black beans. Buy them ready cooked in tins or packets. One cup (170g) contains over 15g of protein and lots of fibre.

Edamame beans make a great addition to salads and stir-fries. A cupful, roughly 150g, contains 17g of protein.

Tofu. This is a great meat substitute, and gives you 18g of protein per 150g serving.

Tempeh is made from fermented soybeans and is something of an acquired taste. But it has more protein than tofu. One serving will deliver almost 25g of protein.

3

The science of keto

The Fast 800 Keto is a keto-based diet (the clue is in the name) but what exactly does that mean? Well, let's start with where you get your day-to-day energy from. Your body works like a hybrid car, able to run on two different fuels: sugar (glucose) and fat. Although protein can be converted into sugar and used as fuel, this is not your body's main priority. It prefers to use the protein in your diet to make hormones, muscles and other essential components to ensure good functioning.

Your body's main go-to fuel is glucose. Glucose is easy for your body to access and provides almost instant energy. If you have to escape from danger, such as an attack by a lion (not very likely these days, but it would have been a bigger problem for our remote ancestors living and foraging on the plains of Africa), then your body will release glucose into your blood so you can run as far and as fast as your legs will carry you.

That said, your sugar stores are relatively limited. You have just 4g (a teaspoonful) of glucose circulating in your blood at any one time.[29]

This amounts to only about 16 calories. And, since

most of us need around 2000 calories a day to sustain us, that won't last long.

Fortunately, you have another 500g of sugar, stored as glycogen, in your liver and muscles. That represents about 2000 calories, so these glycogen stores could keep you going for a while, unless you are exercising heavily. In practice, though, you are unlikely to seriously deplete your glycogen stores because every few hours you probably eat something sugary or with carbs in it, which tops them up.

People often worry that if they don't eat every few hours, they will faint due to lack of energy. But evolution has provided us with body fat as a massive reserve of energy. As far as your body is concerned, the fatty layers you have around your gut are money in the bank, energy stored away for the lean times when you can't find enough to eat (not a big problem for most of us). There are nine calories in a single gram of fat and most of us are carrying around at least 25kg of fat, so those fat stores would provide enough energy to keep us going for ages even if we ate nothing at all.

Most of the time, your body is drawing on a combination of fat and sugar, but it is only when your glucose stores start to run down (because you are fasting, exercising heavily or haven't eaten any carbs for a while) that it switches over to burning fat in a major way.

Your body does this by releasing fatty acids from your fat stores and converting them into chemicals called ketone bodies. These can be used by most cells in your body (including your brain) as fuel.

The process is known as 'flipping the metabolic switch'. It is what your body has evolved to do; so, like a hybrid car going from relying on electricity to using petrol, it should be relatively seamless. But because so many of us are topping up our sugar stores from first thing in the morning till last thing at night, we rarely get to flip the switch, so we rarely do a serious dive into our fat stores.

The idea behind the keto diet is that you cut your consumption of carbs down to such a low level that you drain your glycogen stores and force your body to go into ketone-producing, fat-burning mode. Be warned: unless you are keto adapted (i.e. you have done this before, multiple times), the process can be a little uncomfortable. You will probably feel tired, and may experience 'brain fog'. Some people feel so bad they compare it to a mild case of the flu (which is why they call it 'keto flu'). You may find it hard to exercise – I certainly did. For a few days, everything can feel like a real effort. As you go into ketosis, people may comment that your breath smells 'funny'. Clare says she can always tell when I am in ketosis because my breath smells like nail polish remover.

And then, suddenly, you will start to feel completely different. As you switch into major fat-burning mode, your energy levels soar and your mood lifts. It really does feel like you have suddenly found another gear. This can take a few days, in some cases a bit longer. The more often you do it, the easier it gets.

What is the difference between a low-carb diet and a keto diet?

The main difference between a low-carb and a keto diet is the degree to which you restrict the amount of carbs in your diet. A low-carb diet will typically restrict your carb intake to anywhere between 50g and 150g of carbs a day, which is normally not low enough to induce significant ketosis.

On the first stage of the Fast 800 Keto diet, you reduce your carb consumption to less than 50g a day and, because you also reduce your calories, you will go into ketosis within days. This is surprisingly doable for most people – I will be showing you how in Chapter 4.

The downside of a keto diet is that it can be very restrictive. When you realise that there are nearly 40g of carbs in a baked potato, or a serving of pasta, you can see there are quite a lot of standard foods you will have to avoid.

But the beauty of my Fast 800 Keto plan is that it allows you to gradually add carbs back into your diet as you move through the three stages, so you don't have to torment yourself with the thought that you'll never crunch into a baguette again, or enjoy a roast potato with your Sunday lunch. That's what makes this approach sustainable long-term.

A short history of keto

The term 'keto diet' was first coined by Dr Russell Morse Wilder, a physician based at the Mayo Clinic in the US. Dr Wilder wasn't looking to create a weight loss regime. He was looking for a diet that would help children with epilepsy.

It had been known for more than a thousand years that fasting can help treat epilepsy (as well as other health conditions, like diabetes), but for children fasting was not a practical long-term solution.

So, Dr Wilder decided to see if he could produce the same effect by putting children with epilepsy on a very low-carb diet, one where they would eat just 15g a day, the rest of their calories coming from protein and fat. He called it a keto diet because children, once they started on the diet, started to produce high levels of ketones in their urine. He carried out the first epilepsy trials using his new keto diet more than a hundred years ago, in 1921, and they were a great success.

The keto diet worked so well it remained one of the main ways to treat epilepsy until the discovery of effective drugs. It is still used for people with epilepsy who don't respond to medication. We don't really know why it works, but the combination of low carbs and high fat seem to reduce the 'excitability' of the brain, and therefore the tendency for seizures.

So how and when did a diet aimed at people with epilepsy become a wildly popular way of losing weight? If you go to 'Google trends' and type in the word 'keto diet', you will see that there was very little searching for this term until December 2016, when interest exploded. Some of this is thanks to Dr Dominic D'Agostino, an associate professor at the University of South Florida, and an expert in neuropharmacology. Between 2015 and 2017, he appeared in a number of hugely popular American podcasts, including 'The Joe Rogan Experience' (listened to by over 30 million people worldwide). The main focus of Dr D'Agostino's work is trying to understand how a ketogenic diet protects the brain, and also how it may have a role in protecting people from cancer. He follows a keto diet himself.

Soon after those podcasts went out, Kourtney Kardashian announced that she was 'going keto' and the rest, as they say, is history.

The pros and cons of going keto

Let's start with weight loss, as that is what a lot of people are using it for, and for which it can be extremely effective. A number of studies have shown that when you go into ketosis you feel less hungry, lose weight and shed body fat. This may be due to an effect of ketones on your appetite hormones, your brain or perhaps on your gut microbiota. Most likely, it is a combination of all of these. Other changes that have been seen in short-term trials include rapid falls in cholesterol, blood sugar levels and blood pressure.

The short-term benefits of a keto diet, then, can be

impressive. However, in studies which run for a year or longer, scientists have found that, although short-term results are good, by the end of a year many of those initially allocated to a keto diet are no longer doing it. The problem with standard keto is it can be hard to stick to. When you cut out the carbs you have to anticipate some fairly strong cravings for carb-heavy foods like bread and potatoes.

That is not to say it can't be done. If you have found that a keto diet helps your epilepsy or has reversed your Type 2 diabetes, you may well be able to resist the lure of carbs and find, with time, that your cravings diminish.

Another criticism of keto is that you are encouraged to eat lots of red meat, cream and bacon, which is not only bad for the planet (producing these foods tends to generate a lot of greenhouse gases) but also unlikely to be good for your health, if consumed for a prolonged period.

The answer to this is to modify your diet, make it healthier and more sustainable, by going for keto-friendly foods that are high in healthy fats, like olive oil, avocados, nuts, seeds and fatty fish. This sort of adjustment does make long-term keto an option. But in my view, going keto long-term is not ideal, and is best left to those who benefit from it for health reasons, like epilepsy or Type 2 diabetes.

If you want to lose weight and improve your metabolic health, then, based on lots of studies, I think the best thing you can do is go on a low-calorie keto diet for a limited period to kick-start rapid weight loss; then switch to a more sustainable intermittent fasting pattern, before moving on to a lowish-carb Mediterranean-style diet, a way of eating backed by a huge body of research showing just how good it is for the heart and brain.

Most keto diets don't restrict calories, but my plan does because studies show this is the most effective way to get into ketosis and lose weight, fast. And when it is done in stages, with a gradual introduction of more carbs and calories, the weight loss and other beneficial changes are also more likely to be sustained.

How low is low calorie?

Over the last few years, there have been a number of studies which have looked at the benefits of going on a short-term, very-low-calorie keto diet (VLCKD). Typically, they involve two to three months on very-low-calorie meal replacement shakes (600–800 calories a day). These shakes normally contain less than 50g of carbs and at least 50g of protein a day. After Stage 1, you spend a couple more months upping your carbs and calories and gradually eating more normal food.

A meta-analysis, published in 2020, looked at 12 studies that used this approach and concluded that it is a safe and very effective way to help people who are overweight or obese shed the fat and improve their metabolic health.[30]

Average weight loss among those who stuck to the diet for eight weeks was 15kg, and there were additional impressive reductions in waist size (down by nearly five inches, or 12.6cm), blood sugars, total cholesterol, blood fats and blood pressure. Around 7% of people who started these studies dropped out, which was similar to the drop-out rate in the control groups, who followed a standard low-calorie diet. Side effects were also similar.

Most of these studies were relatively short-term, but one followed patients for two years and, though there was a bit of weight regain, the results were still impressive.[31]

Not only had those who were initially on the VLCKD kept off an average of 12.5kg, after two years, but they had shrunk their waists by almost 11cm and lost three times as much visceral fat as those on a standard low-calorie diet.

The Fast 800 Keto is not as low calorie as some of these programmes. In fact, there are two key differences between the approach used in these VLCKD studies and my plan. First, although you can use meal replacement shakes for some meals if you wish, we encourage you to cook and eat real food, based on our recipes. That way you will be better prepared for when you move to Stage 2 of the diet (which lifts the calorie restriction and reintroduces complex carbohydrates), having built up a repertoire of easy, healthy core meals that you can tweak and add to.

Secondly, we recommend that you do not go as low calorie as is demanded by a VLCKD. On our diet you should aim to eat 800–900 calories a day, and no less than that, because we have found this is enough to effect dramatic weight loss, and to instigate the healthy benefits of fasting, without leaving you feeling so hungry that you struggle to stick to the plan. This is the basis of our menus. And indeed, on hungry days, you can also choose from a range of protein add-ons (see pages 258–61) to help get you through without compromising your weight loss success.

Just to be clear: eating less than 800 calories a day for many weeks counts as a very low-calorie diet (anything over 800 is, technically, a low-calorie diet), and should, ideally, be medically supervised.

But what about starvation mode?

One of the common worries about any diet, particularly one which involves rapid weight loss, is that your body will be so desperate to hold onto its fat that you will go into 'starvation mode'. The fear is that as a result, your metabolic rate, the number of calories your body needs to keep you alive, will fall dramatically, so you end up worse off than you were when you started.

This fear is based, in large part, on the Minnesota Starvation Experiment, a study carried out at the University of Minnesota in the 1940s. For this experiment, a group of young volunteers agreed to go on a semi-starvation diet for 24 weeks, so that scientists could study the impact of this on their bodies and minds.[32]

The volunteers, who were already slim, were kept on a low-calorie diet (around 1500 calories a day), consisting largely of potatoes, turnips, bread and macaroni. This was to mimic the sort of diet being eaten by wartime refugees in Europe. The volunteers lost a lot of weight and the diet had a terrible impact on their mood, with one volunteer getting so depressed he cut off three of his own fingers with an axe. Their metabolic rate crashed, and when they were allowed to eat again, they gorged and gorged.

But, although this experiment is often cited as an example of why you shouldn't diet, what it really demonstrated were the dangers of not eating enough protein. The diet the volunteers were on was incredibly low in fat and protein, so it is not surprising they reacted so badly to it.

Contrary to accepted wisdom, when it comes to weight loss, whether you do it fast or slowly, there is very little evidence that people go into 'starvation mode'. While it is true that when you lose weight your metabolic rate slows down, it is mainly because you are carrying less weight around than you were before you started.

The big question is, does dieting slow your metabolic rate down to an even greater extent than you'd predict, based simply on your weight? This is known as 'metabolic adaptation' and if it happens you will almost certainly find it harder to keep the weight off, long-term.

The answer is, it largely depends on how you lose the weight. Surprisingly enough, while a low-calorie keto diet has been shown to preserve your metabolic rate, a low-fat diet, involving lots of exercise, can lead to some dramatic and what appear to be permanent falls. Let's look at the evidence.

In some of the recent studies in which patients were allocated to a VLCKD, of the sort I described earlier, researchers not only measured changes in weight but also tracked what happened to the patients' metabolic rate. In a recent Spanish trial, for example, where obese patients lost 20kg in four months, researchers measured the patients' metabolic rate at the beginning and end of the study. They found no evidence of 'metabolic adaptation'. In other words the patients' metabolic rate at the end was just what you would predict based on their new weight.

When I made the 'Lose a Stone' series for Channel 4, we found the same thing. We retested our five volunteers six months after their initial dramatic weight loss and not only had they maintained that weight loss but their metabolic rate was exactly what you would expect. There was no sign of metabolic adaptation, let alone 'starvation mode'.

The results of the Biggest Loser Experiment were very different.

The Biggest Loser Experiment

The Biggest Loser was a TV series which ran for many years. It involved very overweight contestants competing to see who could lose the most weight in a short amount of time. They did this by going on a low-fat diet and doing huge amounts of exercise. By the end of each 30-week series, one contestant was crowned the winner. The average weight loss among the successful contestants was around 58kg. But some smart researchers from the National Institute of Diabetes and Digestive and Kidney Diseases wanted to see what happened to them in the long term, particularly to their metabolic rate.[33]

So the scientists measured the weight and metabolic rate of 14 of the contestants at the beginning of the competition, then revisited them six years later.

What they found was that although the contestants had regained most of the weight they'd lost, they had still kept off around 17kg. But the bad news was that since the start of filming, their metabolic rates had fallen dramatically. They were now, on average, burning 500 calories a day less than you would expect for someone of their weight and level of activity. In other words, their metabolic rate had slowed down and stayed down. Why might this be?

No one really knows, but strangely enough there is evidence that if you do lots of exercise your body responds by trying to save energy, and it does this by making your overall metabolic rate fall. This is the opposite of what we've been led to believe.

In a recent study, scientists from the University of Roehampton carefully tracked the calories burnt by more than 1750 volunteers while they were going about their normal lives. Although the volunteers used up more calories while they were exercising, which is what you would expect, their bodies then compensated for this by burning *fewer* calories than normal when they were doing things like sleeping![34]

The scientists found that regular exercise slowed the basal metabolic rate, or BMR (the calories needed to keep their bodies ticking over), of slim people by 28%. The situation was much worse in those who were overweight or obese; in them, only half the calories they burnt while doing exercise translated into real calorie loss at the end of the day. Which means that, far from burning, say, 120 calories every time you run a mile, once you account for the impact that running has on reducing your overall metabolic rate, you are only really burning 60 calories.

All of which sounds rather depressing, but it is actually very liberating. The truth is, you don't have to do lots of exercise to lose weight. I am not going to ask you to take up running or to spend hours at the gym as part of this programme.

Instead, to lose weight, fast, and preserve your metabolic rate, I am going to ask you to start on a keto diet and then slowly build up your activity levels. This will include doing more walking and some resistance exercises, which you can do at home, in just a few minutes. Don't get me wrong. In the long term, becoming more active is a great way to boost your mood, cut your risk of heart disease, stroke and Type 2 diabetes and give your sex life a boost. But, by itself, exercise is not an effective way to lose weight. More on exercise in Chapter 7.

Summary

- The Fast 800 Keto diet is a great way to start your weight loss journey, because you swiftly go into ketosis, and when that happens you start to burn fat, fast.

- Research shows that there are multiple benefits to being on a keto diet, short-term, but the jury is still out about its benefits in the longer term.

- Going keto can certainly be a life-changer if you have epilepsy or Type 2 diabetes, but many people struggle to stick to it. That's why I recommend starting with a low-calorie keto diet, then switching to intermittent fasting, before moving on to a low-carb Med-style diet for long-term weight loss maintenance.

- Remember, by far the best way to lose weight is by changing the way you eat. Exercise is more about fitness and wellbeing. The next chapter goes into much more detail about how to do each stage of the journey.

4

The Fast 800 Keto programme

Now you've read all about the many fantastic reasons to follow the Fast 800 Keto programme, you're probably keen to get started.

If you are familiar with my original Fast 800 programme, some elements of this new regime might seem familiar, but I've introduced a number of important changes, which should make it not only more effective, but much easier to do.

Stage 1: rapid weight loss

The first and most impactful part of the plan is the keto phase, and it's also the simplest. You just need to stick to a low-carb regime of 800–900 calories a day for anything up to 12 weeks. Do this, and you should, at least initially, lose weight at the rate of around 2kg (4lb 6oz) a week (though it will slow down a bit – more on this later).

The combination of low calorie and low carb will ensure that you very rapidly move into ketosis – where you start using your stores of body fat as your main energy source. The first fat to go will be visceral fat, the fat around your tummy, which is also clogging up your internal organs, such as your liver and your pancreas. As that fat disappears, your waist will shrink and your metabolic health will improve. Like the people you'll meet in this book, you should soon see significant improvements in blood pressure, blood sugars and cholesterol, as well as your mood and energy levels. In the first four weeks, you can reasonably expect to lose up to 7kg (a stone), most of it fat.

The easiest way to do the diet is to use our recipes, which are designed to put you into ketosis – fast. They are high in protein and low in carbs, as well as low in calories, and are packed with fibre and nutrients, so you won't go hungry. They are also extremely tasty and very easy to prepare.

That said, if you prefer to make your own meals, that is fine too. The important thing is to ensure you are sticking to the calorie count, while also getting enough protein and not overdoing the carbs. I will give you some tips on how to do this in the next section.

A word on calories

For the Fast 800 diet, we recommended you stick to 800 calories a day on the rapid weight loss phase. But with this diet, you can be a bit more relaxed about your calorie intake – eating 800–900, and even on the odd day up to 1000 calories. This is because the combination of restricting your calories with going very low carb/keto will put you into ketosis even if you are taking in slightly more food.

This does not mean you can go mad. Our meal plans at the back of the book offer you daily menus adding up to between 800 and 900 calories. But we want you to feel free on some days to add small amounts of high-protein/high-fat, keto-friendly add-ons, such as a spoonful of Greek yoghurt, a stick of cheese, some extra tofu or nuts (see add-on options on pages 258–261). In our view, including a healthy add-on is far, far better than giving into a craving and reaching for a pastry, a chocolate bar or a packet of crisps.

Low carb does not mean no carb

Although this initial phase is very low carb, it is not no carb. On the Fast 800 Keto, we recommend you enjoy carbs in the most filling and nutritious form possible – in vegetables, and in small quantities of complex carbs such as chickpeas and pulses, nuts and seeds, all of which are built into the recipes.

And, because the nutritional benefits of salads and green leafy vegetables massively outweigh any downsides of adding a few extra calories or carbs, we believe you should pile your plate high with them in all three stages of the Fast 800 Keto plan. Drizzling them with a little extra-virgin olive oil is fine, too. These are all keto-friendly foods.

Remember, to achieve ketosis you have to stop feeding your body carbs that can be easily converted into sugar in the blood. Which means, for this stage of the diet, all bread, cereals, cakes, biscuits, pasta and potatoes are off the table, out of the house or given to the neighbours.

We also recommend you avoid starchy vegetables and most fruit (apart from berries, which are not only a great source of nutrients, but also packed with fibre, so, when eaten in small quantities, can be digested more slowly without compromising your body's ketogenic state). Unfortunately, a biscuit or a small bar of chocolate could be enough to tip your body out of ketosis and back into sugar-burning mode.

The Rule of 50

Whichever approach you decide on – following our recipes or designing your own – you need to keep a close eye on your 'macros', that is, the amount of protein and carbs you are consuming.

During the rapid weight loss stage of the diet, you are aiming to consume at least 50g of protein a day, but to keep your daily carb intake at less than 50g. I call it the Rule of 50.

The meal plans at the back of the book have been carefully calibrated to achieve this. Our recipes also show you, at a glance, how many grams of protein and how many grams of carbs there are in any given dish. If you're going it alone and making your own dishes, as long as you know the Rule of 50, it shouldn't be too difficult to work out your own menu plan. Just check the protein and carb content on the packaging of any given item, or look it up online (e.g. one chicken breast is 31g of protein per 100g, a 100g tin of tuna contains 28g of protein). Don't feel too worried if you are slightly out on any given day – you just need to aim for an average <50g carbs and >50g protein over a typical week.

Protein in every meal, but not to excess

The reason we are keener than ever that you have plenty of protein on your plate *every* time you eat is that, as I explained in Chapter 2, protein is a key driver of hunger and, unlike fat and carbs, it is not stored by your body. So making sure you have decent levels of high-quality protein will not only help you to maintain your muscle mass but also keep your appetite suppressed. However, a word of caution. In Stage 1, you also have to put limits on how much protein you eat, because if you eat much more than you need your body will convert any excess into sugar (by a process called gluconeogenesis), which could sabotage your attempts to go into ketosis. It is a balancing act.

As you transition to Stages 2 and 3, you will be increasing your daily protein intake. Later in this chapter, I will explain how.

Two meals or three?

Throughout each phase of the Fast 800 Keto plan, you get to choose whether you prefer two meals a day or three. Many people find having two slightly larger meals each day is more convenient and satisfying than three smaller meals. One popular pattern is having a late breakfast, skipping lunch, then eating an early evening meal. Try the different approaches and see what works for you.

The advantage of going for two meals like this is that you are doing Time-Restricted Eating (TRE), a form of intermittent fasting in which you eat your day's meals within a narrower time window. This is a great way of boosting the impact of ketosis, and the evidence for its general health benefits is growing.

The original TRE studies were on rats, and it took a while for human studies to get going. In fact, I was involved with one of the first human TRE studies, carried out by Dr Jonathan Johnston of the University of Surrey.[35]

For this study, which was published in 2018 in the *Journal of Nutritional Sciences*, he recruited 16 healthy volunteers and measured their body fat, blood sugar and cholesterol levels. They were then randomly assigned to TRE or a control group.

The TRE people were asked to stick to their normal diet but to move their breakfast 90 minutes later, and their dinner time 90 minutes earlier. This meant that for three extra hours each day they were without food (i.e. fasting). Everyone kept a food and sleep diary to ensure they were eating the same amount as normal.

Ten weeks later, they repeated the tests. They found that the group who had eaten breakfast later and dinner earlier had, on average, each lost around 1.6kg of body fat. They had also seen bigger falls in blood sugar and cholesterol than the control group.

A more recent study did something similar. This time, researchers took 19 overweight volunteers with metabolic syndrome (raised blood sugar, blood pressure and cholesterol) and asked them to eat within a 10-hour window (i.e. a form of TRE known as 14:10). Although the recruits were asked to eat as much as normal, many of them said they were eating less, due to the shorter eating window. Extending their overnight fast also led to a significant reduction in body fat, blood pressure and total cholesterol. Blood sugar and insulin levels also improved.[36]

At the back of the book, you'll see a series of meal plans offering you a choice of two or three meals a day. Either way, you can be confident all your nutrients will have been calculated for you, and your total calories for the day will have added up to between 800 and 900. Add as many non-starchy vegetables as you like.

What about meal replacement shakes?

Although it is preferable, as explained in Chapter 3, to try to cook most meals from scratch, meal replacement shakes can be very helpful because you don't have to worry about counting calories for every single meal. They are particularly helpful when you are dashing out first thing in the morning, or you need something to take to work for lunch.

Our range of shakes, available at thefast800.com, come in a variety of flavours, are very low in carbs and contain plenty of high-quality protein, as well as decent amounts of fibre.

You buy them in 500g packets, which each provide 10 meals. A 50g shake – made up of five scoops of powder mixed with 300ml water – provides 199 calories, and makes a surprisingly filling breakfast, lunch or evening meal, containing 22g of good-quality protein, 7g of fibre and just 5g of carbs, as well as a quarter of all your daily vitamin and mineral needs.

Instead of water, you can mix the shake powders with a cup of almond milk. This gives it a creamier texture, a bit more protein and fibre, very few carbs (1.8g) and adds just 39 calories. Unfortunately, you can't use cow's milk because it is far more calorific and contains lots of natural sugars.

Using keto sticks

When you start the Fast 800 Keto, it is likely to take four or five days, perhaps a little longer, for your body to go into ketosis, and you will be understandably keen to find out when the magic moment happens.

One of the best ways of keeping an eye on your progress is by using keto strips. These are thin strips of plastic with an active agent on one end, and are cheap and easy to use. You can buy them online, or in pharmacies. They come with full instructions, but basically you dip the end of the strip into your urine stream or into a clean container holding a fresh sample of your urine, and then compare any colour change with a colour chart on the side of the packet. The darker the colour, the higher your ketone levels. You are aiming for what is called 'nutritional ketosis', where the strips are telling you that you are in 'small' or 'moderate' ketosis, not 'large' ketosis.

These strips were originally created for people with Type 1 diabetes, to detect diabetic ketoacidosis, a dangerous and potentially life-threatening condition. This is very different from nutritional ketosis, and happens when your body isn't capable of producing enough insulin to bring your blood sugars down. This should not happen on a keto diet, but if your ketone levels are registering as very high, you might want to introduce a few more carbs into your diet.

You can also measure your ketone levels by pricking your finger and testing your blood, or using a keto breathalyser; but these methods are more expensive.

I found using keto strips, while doing the diet, was enormously motivating, and that's what lots of other people have told me. It is genuinely exciting seeing the strips change colour and a surprisingly useful deterrent if you are tempted by a biscuit. (I remember thinking to myself, 'If I eat that biscuit then I will no longer be in a state of ketosis and I won't be seeing a colour change next time I go to the loo. How disappointing that would be'.)

Becoming more active

Although many people will be turning to the Fast 800 Keto to lose weight fast – and this is the best possible way to do that! – your main goal should be to improve your overall health. Losing weight is good, but being more active is very important too. I am not asking you to run a marathon (which would be an extremely bad idea while on a rapid weight loss diet) but everyone on this plan benefits significantly from increasing their activity levels.

As I will show you in Chapter 7, by combining resistance and aerobic exercises with a higher-protein diet, you will be improving your aerobic fitness, as well as preserving your muscle mass.

Just as important, becoming more active will boost your mood and improve your sleep (you will find more on this in Chapter 6). All of which will keep you on track when it comes to following the diet, and will also help you maintain weight loss, long-term.

How long should I stick to Stage 1?

This very much depends on your reasons for following the diet and how you feel on it. If you are only carrying a few kilos of excess weight, or you want to get your eating habits back on track after a holiday or a period of indulgence, then a few weeks on Stage 1 might be enough. But if you have been warned that your blood sugar levels are too high, if you have Type 2 diabetes, or if you have quite a bit of weight to lose, it is safe for you to stay on Stage 1 for longer, but no more than 12 weeks. Although people have stayed on 800-calorie-a-day diets for longer than 12 weeks, they are normally under medical supervision.

Once you have decided it is time to move on, you can switch to Stage 2 and continue to lose weight, though more slowly. Be warned that when you first come off a strict keto diet you typically put on a bit of weight, almost all of it water. That's because, as your glycogen sugar stores rebuild, they trap water. So, expect the numbers on the scales to stand still for a while, or even rise a bit. You will still feel good and your waist won't suddenly expand, but the numbers probably won't go on falling at the rate you have got used to.

The other point worth repeating is that this programme is really flexible and you can, of course, skip Stage 2 and go straight to Stage 3, which is the long-term weight maintenance phase, designed to keep your weight stable. Again, expect a temporary weight blip as your body takes on more water. Switching over (and switching back) can be done at any time that suits you.

Stage 2: intermittent fasting

For Stage 2 of the Fast 800 Keto, I recommend that you follow, at least initially, a 3:4 plan. This means being strict with yourself, sticking to your 'fasting days' of 800–900 calories a day on a very low-carb diet on four days a week (Monday to Thursday), and then taking a more relaxed approach over the weekend: eating normally, without counting calories, but adding in more protein and more complex carbs, and generally being careful.

This is a popular form of intermittent fasting. In previous books (such as *The Fast 800*), I have written extensively about the science behind intermittent fasting, so I won't go into it in great depth here. The basic idea is that you cut your calories a few days a week (if it's four days, then it is 3:4; if it is two days then it is 5:2), and otherwise eat normally. You still lose weight, albeit more slowly than on the rapid weight loss stage; you still switch on your body's reboot and repair mechanisms; and you will get health benefits from continuing to regularly flip the metabolic switch, going between burning sugar and burning fat. (If you are interested in learning more about the benefits of intermittent fasting, I recommend an article written by one of my scientific heroes, Professor Mark Mattson, and published in the *New England Journal of Medicine* – 'Effects of intermittent fasting on health, ageing and disease' – which provides an excellent summary of some of the latest research and is available, free, online.)[37]

The 3:4 plan

The 3:4 approach is based on feedback from the more than 44,000 people who have done our online Fast 800 programme. Many of them, after doing really well on Stage 1, have felt nervous about going straight on to 5:2, where you stick to 800 calories two days a week. This seemed like too big a step. So we have introduced 3:4 as an option, and the feedback has been excellent. It is what Adrian and Katie from 'Lose a Stone' did (see pages 13 and 112); it is also what Curtis still does (see page 124). They, and others, have found this 3:4 pattern fits best into their busy working lives.

If you stick to a keto diet during the week, and add more protein and carbs at the weekend (and even the occasional alcoholic drink), you will be doing what is known as 'keto cycling', regularly flipping the metabolic switch and going in and out of ketosis. This is what our bodies evolved to do naturally and the more you do it the easier it gets. Research done with male athletes has shown that, as well as being a stepping-stone from full-on keto to something that is more sustainable long-term, keto cycling leads to more muscle growth, higher levels of testosterone and better performance when combined with resistance exercises.[38]

Upping your carbs and protein

On the three days a week when you are not being so strict with your calories, we recommend you move to eating a healthy, Mediterranean-style diet, one that includes more carbs (somewhere between 50 and 120g a day) and more protein.

The carbs you add in should be fibre-rich 'complex carbohydrates' (so called because the body metabolises them slowly), including root vegetables (carrots, butternut squash, sweet potato), wholegrains, lentils and beans. You can occasionally include a slice of brown seeded or sourdough bread, a healthy dessert or a piece of fruit. At the end of many of the recipes in this book you'll see we have also included 'non-fast day' options with suggestions for healthy protein 'add-ons', such as a tablespoonful of Greek yoghurt, some cheese, or a handful of edamame beans. Some recipes allow you to double the size of your portions.

Incidentally, key to the success of this stage of the diet is keeping your fasting days consecutive, so your body has a chance to go into ketosis and stay there. Your body will swiftly adapt to this new regime and you will find that you flick in and out of ketosis each week without any difficulty and without experiencing side effects, like keto flu. You will also find your cravings have diminished, which means you will find it easier to avoid sugary foods and processed carbs.

Adding in Time-Restricted Eating (TRE)

For Stage 2, if you haven't already done so, we encourage you to introduce an element of TRE.

I recommend establishing a pattern you can comfortably manage, long-term. Start with 12:12 (which means fasting for 12 hours and eating within a 12-hour window each day – for instance between 8am and 8pm), but aim to widen your fasting window if you can.

The easiest way to start is to aim to stop eating at least three hours before bed, and then not eat again until at least an hour after you wake up. You can obviously drink water and a splash of milk in tea or coffee is fine, but don't overdo it.

In the evenings, when you have stopped eating, you can have as many calorie-free drinks as you want – water, herbal teas, etc – but, obviously, no alcohol!

When to move on to Stage 3

The obvious answer to this is when you reach your target weight or have reached whatever other goal you may have set yourself. However, be aware that if you are trying to reverse Type 2 diabetes, you should be aiming to lose at least 10% of your body weight, and you should continue dieting *even if your blood sugars return to normal before you achieve that amount of weight loss*. This is because lower blood sugar levels do not in themselves necessarily mean that you have fully reversed your Type 2 and got your pancreas back on track. Professor Roy Taylor (who is leading the field with research on reversing Type 2 diabetes through rapid weight loss) has shown that the pancreas can take up to a year to fully recover.

Some people find that, rather than suddenly moving from Stage 2 to Stage 3, it works better to gradually increase the amount of carbs in their diet until their weight loss starts to slow. At this point they know they have reached their own personal carb threshold – i.e. the amount of carbs they can safely eat before they start to put on weight again. Everyone's threshold is different. It can be high, or it can be low. But it can only be judged by trial and error. Knowing our threshold is a useful step towards maintaining a healthy weight for life.

Stage 3: the long-term maintenance plan

This stage is about going back to normal eating, but not to the way you used to eat before. Do that and you will undermine all the hard work you have done. Instead, I would suggest that you move on to a relatively low-carb, high-protein Med-style diet, which is the most effective way not only to keep the weight off long-term, but also to reduce your risk of heart disease, cancer, Type 2 diabetes and dementia. It is a way of eating that has been shown to reduce depression and anxiety, as well as improve sleep.

Research shows that if you stick to a lowish-carb Med-style diet – to recap: one which includes plenty of oily fish, nuts, olive oil, vegetables, legumes, yoghurt and fruit, and modest amounts of complex carbs, such as brown rice, lentils and beans – you can stop counting calories and will not regain the weight you have so diligently lost, while still enjoying the occasional glass of wine or slice of cake.

This is how I live my life. Unlike my wife, Clare, I am not naturally slim. I have to keep an eye on my weight and my waist, or I would balloon. By sticking to a healthy Med-style diet, and doing the odd fasting day to compensate if I have overindulged or I feel my trousers pinching, I manage to keep my weight, waist, blood sugars and blood pressure down, without calorie counting. You will find much more on how to follow a Med-style diet in Chapter 6.

Upping your protein further

Now that you are not on a calorie-restricted phase of the diet, you should increase your protein levels again. Ideally, you should now be eating 1g of protein per kilo of your body weight. In other words, if you are 80kg, like me, by Stage 3 you should be eating between 80 and 120g of protein a day, which is considerably more than you will have been doing in Stage 1.

If you eat a couple of eggs for breakfast, that is 12g of protein. A smallish bit of fish for lunch with some lentils is around 30g, and if you have grilled chicken and veggies for your evening meal that is another 40g. All of which takes you above 80g for the day.

Eating more protein keeps me on the straight and

narrow – it means my muscles and bones have the amino acids they need, and I'm much less likely to be tempted by cravings.

Keeping the weight off long-term

Many people believe that long-term weight loss is next to impossible; I have heard over and over again that 99% of diets fail and that people who go on them end up as fat, if not fatter, than when they started. I'm not sure what the origin of this myth is, but it may be a study published in 1957 in which 100 people with obesity were put on a diet and two years later 98 of them had put on most or all of the weight they had lost.

There are lots of crazy diets out there, many promoted by celebrities, and most of them will undoubtedly fail. But even a cursory read through recent research will show you that if you follow a decent diet (one which has some science behind it), there is a good chance you will keep some, or most, of that weight off. And, contrary to what many people believe, rapid weight loss diets can be more effective in the short, medium and long term.

That's because losing weight, fast, is very motivating and many studies have shown that the amount of weight that you lose in the first four weeks of a diet is a powerful predictor of how you will do, long-term.

A meta-analysis by American researchers looked at dozens of studies in which standard advice had been compared with a rapid weight loss approach, and where they had followed participants for up to five years. The researchers found that people following a rapid weight loss approach were more successful 'at all years of follow-up'. At the five-year follow-up, they found that 58% of men and 48% of women had kept off at least 5% of their body weight, which is enough to make a big difference in terms of health.[39]

In the next two chapters, you will read a lot more about how to plan for and follow the different stages of this diet, and, crucially, how to turn the core principles of the programme into a way of life.

The Fast 800 Keto at a glance

	How to fast	What to eat
Stage 1 Rapid weight loss	800–900 cals a day for up to 12 weeks, with the possibility of protein add-ons taking you up to 1000 cals when needed.	Real food (see recipes) or meal replacement shakes, based on eating more than 50g protein and less than 50g carbs a day.

	How to fast	What to eat
Stage 2 Intermittent fasting: the 3:4 or the 5:2	800–900 cals, a few days a week (ideally on consecutive days), taking a more relaxed approach on non-fasting days; and adding in TRE.	On fast days: real food (see recipes) or shakes. On non-fast days: Med-style diet, upping your protein to 60–80g and practising some portion control.
Stage 3 Maintenance	No calorie counting, though you need to keep an eye on your weight and waist.	Healthy Med-style diet, with more protein than before: 90–100g a day for men, 70–80g for women.

WHAT DOES AN 800-900 CALORIE DAY LOOK LIKE?

Cheesy Asparagus Prosciutto Bites
Keto Pancakes with Yoghurt and Berries
Steamed Fish with Tomato and Pepper Sauce
Raspberry Fool
Total for the day = 844 kcals / 49g protein

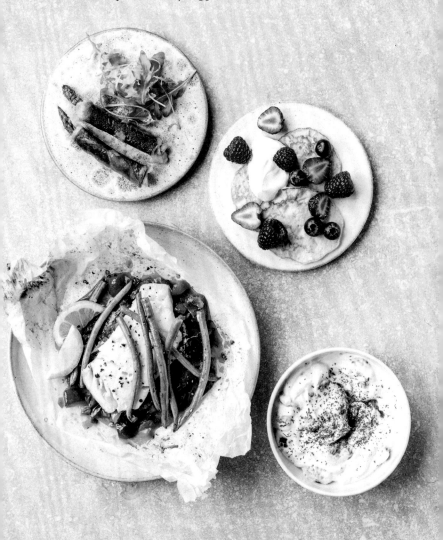

Rapid Bircher with Apple and Cinnamon
Pea and Mint Soup with Feta Add-On
Pulled Pork with Cider Vinegar and Honey
Total for the day = 885 kcals / 51g protein

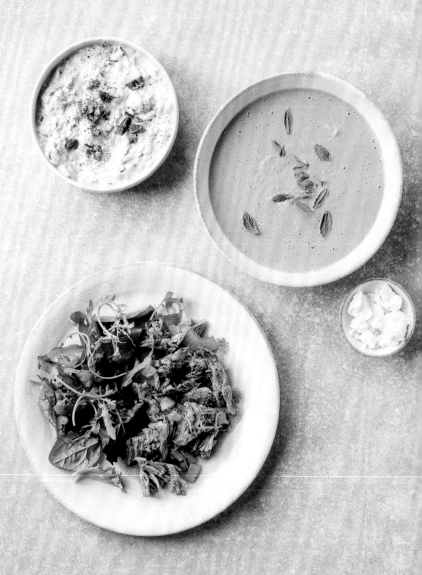

Scrambled Eggs with Smoked Salmon,
   Feta and Avocado with Mixed Seeds Add-On
Goat's Cheese Frittata with Greens and Diced Figs
Black Bean Chilli with Cabbage Pappardelle
Total for the day = 848 kcals / 50.2g protein

Spinach and Ham Omelette
Curried Smoked Haddock Chowder
Speedy One Pan Thai Red Curry with Salmon
Total for the day = 830 kcals / 73.5g protein

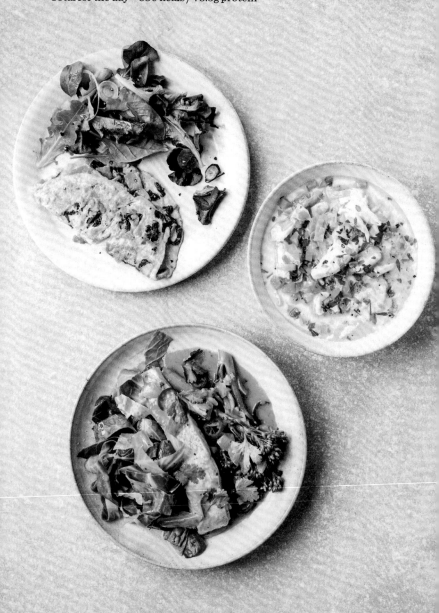

Cheese and Chive Muffins
Protein Wrap with Smoked Salmon, Cream Cheese and Capers
Aubergine Parmigiana with Lentils
Total for the day = 895 kcals / 53g protein

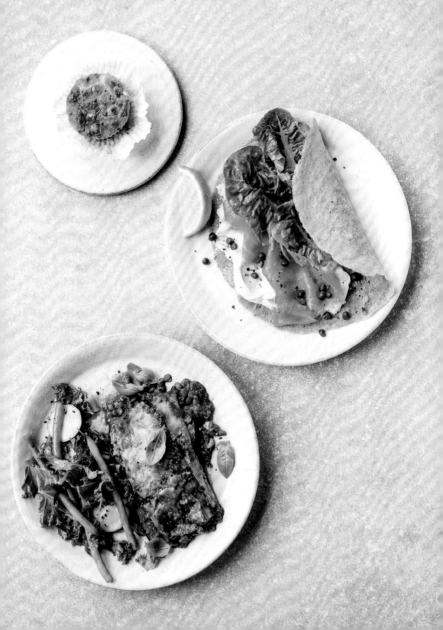

Tandoori Chicken Kebabs with Raita
Tuscan Lamb Stew with White Beans
Dark Choc Bites
Total for the day = 811 kcals / 72.2g protein

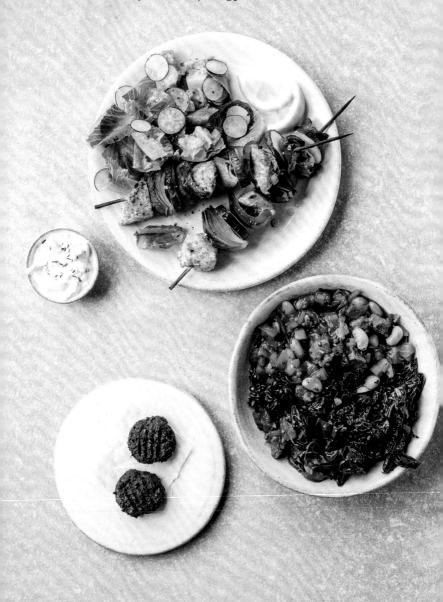

Easy Chicken, Spinach and Tomato Soup
Prawn Curry with Coconut Milk with Edamame Beans Add-On
Total for the day = 841 kcals / 58.5g protein

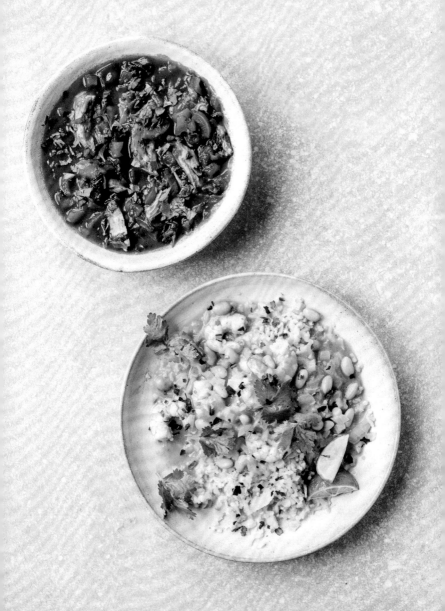

Breakfast Traybake
Protein Salad with Tuna, Roasted Red Peppers,
**   Edamame and Harissa**
Total for the day = 797 kcals / 52g protein

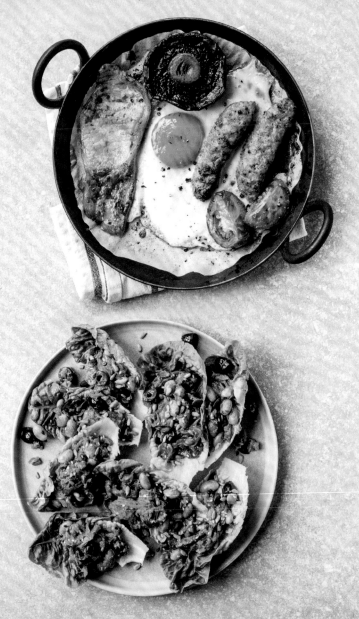

5

It's all in the preparation

As you will have gathered from the outline of the Fast 800 Keto programme in the previous chapter, the initial rapid weight loss stage will represent a short, sharp change to your current eating and drinking lifestyle. In my experience, you are far more likely to be successful if you take a bit of time to plan for how you are going to manage it in advance. This really is important. As the great Benjamin Franklin, scientist, diplomat and one of the founding fathers of the United States, eloquently put it, 'By failing to prepare, you are preparing to fail.' Here are some of the key things that you would be wise to do before you start.

Speak to your doctor

If you have any concerns about your health, or if you have a lot of weight to lose (anything over 2 stone, or 15kg), it's a good idea to talk to your GP or a health professional before starting on the Fast 800 Keto plan. This is particularly important if you are taking medication, as the dramatic changes in body composition that are very likely to result from being on this diet might affect the dosage of any medication you are on.

If you have Type 2 diabetes, your blood sugar levels will come down, often within days, so if you are on medication you will need a plan in place for reducing it accordingly.

If you have high blood pressure, losing weight may mean you are able to reduce or even come off tablets completely. I'd advise getting a home blood pressure measuring kit. If you start feeling dizzy it can be a sign that you are over-medicated. Your GP should be happy to help monitor your progress and work with you to taper off your medicines as and when appropriate.

My hope is that most doctors will be delighted that you are taking responsibility for your own health but some might not approve of rapid weight loss. If so, point out that recent studies show rapid weight loss can be *more* successful than slower methods, long-term. If you think it is helpful, do print out or offer to email your GP links to key research which you can find at https://thefast800.com/health-professionals/.

Those of you with Type 2 diabetes might also suggest your doctor look at a link on the Newcastle University website, which includes a factsheet for doctors written by Professor Roy Taylor (one of the UK's leading diabetes specialists).[40]

I know a lot of doctors who have themselves followed earlier versions of my Fast 800 plan, lost lots of weight and now recommend it to their patients.

Having said that, we don't recommend this diet

plan if you are under 18, underweight, have a history of eating disorders, are pregnant or breastfeeding, have a significant psychiatric disorder or medical condition, including epilepsy and gallstones, or are on certain medications. It is also not appropriate if you are recovering from surgery, or if you are generally frail.

Clear the decks

I'm the first to admit that when it comes to sweet treats, I have almost zero willpower, and I find that, in the words of Oscar Wilde, once I have been tempted, 'The only way to get rid of the temptation is to yield to it. Resist it, and your soul grows sick with longing for the things it has forbidden to itself.'

The truth is that willpower is hugely overrated and relying on it is one of the main reasons why so many diets fail. If you've spent years eating whatever you like, whenever you like, your old habits are likely to be hard to break.

You have to create an environment in which it is easier to succeed than to fail. This may mean changing your route to work, your kids' school or the gym to avoid passing your favourite coffee shop where you buy your frothy coffee and muffin (a cappuccino and muffin easily add up to 500 calories). And it almost certainly means clearing your house of tantalisingly tempting junk food and 'treats'. These include cakes, biscuits and sugary breakfast cereals, as well as crisps and other savoury snacks. I want you also to keep clear of alcohol, at least for the first month, so whether you pour your booze down the sink, give it to your friends or put it in a cupboard, out of sight, is up to you.

For me, it is relatively easy to steer clear of temptation as our children are grown up and have all left home and my wife, Clare, does not have a sweet tooth. But what do you do if your partner insists on keeping biscuits in the house and eating crisps in front of you? Or if your kids say, 'I'm starving' as soon as they get back from school, and complain about the lack of snacks?

This is a tough one, and your best bet is to try and get your friends and family on board with what you are doing. The research shows that people do better if they do it as a couple, and I have seen countless cases where because one person decided to give the diet a go, other members of the family joined in and were amazed by the changes.

As for the kids, well, they really don't need to be eating junk food any more than you do, and by removing ultra-processed foods from the house you will be doing them a favour, long-term. If you learn healthy eating habits when you are a child, you are far more likely to be eating healthily when you are an adult. Plus, you are creating a healthy microbiome for the future.

When I was a child, we were allowed sweets once a week, which we went out to buy at the local shop, and we only had biscuits or crisps as a special treat.

If you find this is too challenging, then all I can suggest is that you put all the junk in one cupboard and either lock it and give the key to your partner, or put a large skull and crossbones on the door and hope that will deter you. Remember, this diet is not forever; the key rapid weight loss stage is for 12 weeks, or less, and within a few weeks your cravings for junk should begin to fade.

Stock up with the healthy stuff

Once you have emptied your cupboards and fridge of any tempting junk foods, it is time to fill these spaces with the healthy stuff. Take a look at the recipes at the back of this book and decide what you are going to eat during the first week of the diet, and write a list of the foods you are going to have to buy. You might want to practise a few recipes before the diet itself begins, just to reassure yourself that they are tasty and filling.

If you have to travel, or go to work, you may also want to plan, well in advance, what foods you can cook and take with you.

In the keto phase of the diet, you are going to be eating plenty of healthy protein (fish, meat, tofu, etc). You will also be allowed generous amounts of leafy green vegetables of all kinds (spinach, kale, cabbage, broccoli, cauliflower, Brussels sprouts) and salad basics (lettuce, rocket, endive, cucumber, tomatoes, pepper), drizzled with olive oil. You will need some nuts for the occasional snack, and do stock up on eggs as, besides being one of our favourite protein-rich breakfasts, a boiled egg makes a satisfying high-protein, low-carb, low-calorie snack.

It is important that you try the recipes and cook from scratch as much as you can, but there will always be moments when you simply don't have time for this. In those circumstances, having a supply of low-carb, high-protein meal replacement shakes to hand can be invaluable. I've tried a lot of meal replacement shakes and unfortunately most not only taste horrible but are also surprisingly high in carbs. That's why we created the Fast 800 range of shakes, which are all keto-friendly. If you fancy trying them out, they are available on our website.

Record 'before' and 'after' measurements

You may encounter bumps along the road on this diet, and even find you enter weight loss plateaus, so keeping 'before' and 'after' measurements is vital for showing you how far you have come, and for occasionally reminding yourself why you are doing this. Do make sure to write them down, either in the chart on pages 276–77 of this book, on your phone or somewhere accessible.

Weigh yourself
Before you begin, I want you to weigh yourself and work out your Body Mass Index (there are plenty of online calculators that will do this for you). If you identify as White, then a BMI of 25 or over is considered 'overweight', while a BMI of 30 or over is considered 'obese'. But if you are from a Black, Asian or Hispanic

ethnic background these numbers are going to be lower.

In China and Japan, for example, you are considered overweight if your BMI is 24 or more and obese if it is 28 or higher. In India, they are even less generous. You are considered overweight with a BMI of 23 or more, and obese with a BMI of 27 or over.

That's because, as we saw with Adrian, if you have an Asian ethnic background you are far more likely to develop Type 2 diabetes, heart disease or hypertension than someone who identifies as White with the same BMI.[41]

Measure your waist

BMI has its critics, not least because you can be slim and very muscular and still have a high BMI. This is not a problem for most of us, but since we know that *where* you store your fat is as important as how much you are carrying, I do recommend you also measure your waist.

To do it properly, you first find the top of your hip and the bottom of your ribs, then put a tape measure midway between those points. It should be just above your belly button. Breathe out naturally before taking the measurement – don't hold your tummy in! Make sure it's reasonably tight, but isn't digging into your skin.

You are measuring your waist because it is a good way of estimating your levels of visceral fat, the fat which collects in your tummy and infiltrates your internal organs when there is no more room to store it under your skin, and which in turn is linked to metabolic syndrome.

Visceral fat is the fat I want you to lose. Broadly

speaking, you can expect to lose 1cm off your waistline for every kilo you lose, so the changes you see with the tape measure will be much slower than those you see on the scales. Try to measure your waist every couple of weeks (at the same time each day) just to check you are moving in the right direction.

According to the British Heart Foundation, if you are a man, a waist size below 94cm (37in) is considered low risk, while above that is high risk. For women, low risk is below 80cm (31.5in), high risk is 80–88cm (31.5–34.6in) and more than 88cm (34.6in) is considered very high.

But if you are ethnically African Caribbean, South Asian, Chinese or Japanese, the numbers are lower. For men, a waist size below 90cm (35.4in) is low risk, while women have to be below 80cm (31.5in) to be considered low risk, and anything above is very high risk.

According to the most recent surveys, in the UK an alarming 80% of middle-aged women and 70% of middle-aged men have a waist measurement which puts them in the 'high' or 'very high' risk categories.

If you don't have a tape measure, another simple way to measure your waist is to do the 'string test'. You get some string, cut it to your height, fold it in half, then see if it fits around your tummy. Your waist should, ideally, be less than half your height. I am 180cm tall, so I try to keep my waist below 90cm.

Test your blood pressure
Raised blood pressure – hypertension – is a common

but hidden disease. A third of British adults are hypertensive, rising to half of those over 65 (I am 64). All the contributors we tested for my TV series, 'Lose a Stone', had raised blood pressure before beginning the programme.

High blood pressure puts a strain on your blood vessels, your heart and other organs, including your brain and kidneys. But unless you've been tested you won't know if you have a problem because there are rarely any symptoms. The first warning may be when you have a heart attack or stroke.

I feel passionately about the dangers posed by raised blood pressure because two close male friends – both of whom were younger than me – have died as a result of untreated hypertension. I also have a strong family history of heart attacks and strokes, so I know that I am at increased risk.

That's why I keep a portable blood pressure monitor at home (you can buy them for less than £20 from a chemist or online) and test myself at least once a month.

Your blood pressure is a measure of how hard your heart has to work to drive blood around your body. Mine hovers around 125/75, depending on the time of day and how stressed I am feeling. When I put on weight (as I did on the ultra-processed food diet I wrote about earlier), it shot up to 145/95, which is very unhealthy. The NHS says an ideal blood pressure is between 90/60 and 120/80 – you're considered to have high blood pressure if your reading is 140/90 or higher.

The good news is that if you are hypertensive your blood pressure should start to come down within weeks of starting the Fast 800 Keto programme. If you can reduce your systolic blood pressure (that is the larger number) by 10 points, you cut your risk of having a stroke by 33% and your risk of a heart attack by 20%.[42]

But I repeat: if you are on blood pressure medication you must talk to your doctor before starting the programme, so they can adjust your medication if necessary. Otherwise, there is a danger that you will feel dizzy due to being over-medicated.

Take a photo

Before you start the diet, take a selfie or get a friend to take a photo of you. Keep this somewhere safe so you can compare the outward changes. You will want to show people the 'before' and 'after' in a few weeks' time and you'll kick yourself if you haven't got photographic evidence.

Your 'before' picture should also help you resist temptation when you find yourself standing outside a bakery looking longingly at the pies. Before you go in, remember that picture, and all the aches and pains that came with it; instead, give an approving nod to your strong, slimmer reflection in the window, throw back your shoulders and walk on by.

Keep a diary

Along with recording things like weight, waist and blood pressure, I recommend you keep a dedicated notebook or have somewhere on your phone to jot down how you are feeling, as well as ideas for recipes or tricks that work for you, and any that don't. Whatever you think might prove useful.

It is also a good idea to write down the main reasons why you want to lose weight. There will be times over the coming weeks and months when you will experience moments of doubt and be tempted to stop and go back to your old ways of living and eating, so it is important to clearly set out your goals somewhere you can flick back to whenever you feel a wobble coming on.

Garner support

If you want to maximise your chances of weight loss success, it is essential you tell your friends and family about your plans and your reasons for doing it. Making a public commitment like this means you are more likely to stick to it, and you never know, someone might want to join you on the programme – then you can buddy up and keep each other going.

If people know you are on this diet, they are more likely to be considerate about what they eat around you and less likely to offer you 'treat' foods or put temptation your way. Encourage them to try out the recipes with you – they don't have to stick to 800 calories per day (many of the recipes have tips for how to adapt them for non-fast days), but the more you can do together, the better.

Studies show that being part of a group – even if it's just you and one friend, a fasting buddy – will significantly improve your chances of success. You can also join thefast800.com community, where you will get lots of professional support.

Decide when to start!

You've bought this book, so you are obviously keen to lose weight. All you need to do now is decide when. Choose a time when you can focus on it for at least two weeks without too many distractions. It's fine to keep working; in fact, keeping busy will help, but better to have a period with fewer pressing social engagements. You don't want your 50th birthday or a friend's wedding to derail you just as you get into the swing of things. That said, I know quite a few 'mothers of the bride' (and some fathers) who have decided they need to go on this diet to get in shape for the big day.

Summary

- If you are frail, have a medical condition or are on medication, do see a health professional before starting. And visit thefast800.com to see if you are suitable for this approach.

- Measure your weight and your waist and use home test kits to measure your blood pressure, so you can see the before and after changes.

- Clear the junk food out of your cupboards.

- Read the recipes at the back of this book, plan what you are going to eat during the first week and buy the necessary ingredients. You might want to practise cooking some of the meals in advance.

- Tell your friends and loved ones what you are doing and get their support.

6

The diet in practice: how to stay on track

So, you've done the preparation. You've decided on your goals, restocked the cupboards, told your friends and family. Above all, you know why you are doing this diet, how important it is for your health and happiness. This chapter is all about what the diet feels like in practice; what to expect at each stage; and how to stay motivated when you are struggling, or your weight plateaus, or simply when life gets in the way. I will be offering you lots of tips and advice on how to build a sustainable routine, as well as inspirational stories from other Fast 800 Keto dieters, to help you stay on track.

Stage 1: what to expect

How you'll feel in the first two weeks

I won't lie: it's not easy to cut your calorie intake right back, when your body (and brain) have spent most of your life eating so much more. You're going to have to go through a process of adjustment – but it is *so* going to be worth it!

The first week or two are likely to be tough as your body adapts to fewer calories and to flipping the metabolic switch, to burning fat rather than sugar. The best way to minimise 'carb withdrawal' is by drinking lots and lots of water. Tap water is fine, but it will probably be more enjoyable if you keep a jug cooled in the fridge. A few slices of lemon will also jazz it up. Any time you feel tempted to eat a snack, have a glass of cold water and wait 10 minutes. I promise you, the cravings will pass.

Aim to drink a big glass of water when you wake up in the morning, a big glass mid-morning and a glass with each meal. Black tea, herbal tea and coffee are a good distraction, if you do feel hungry, but try not to have more than four cups of coffee a day, as it may interfere with your sleep and push up your blood pressure. If you want a splash of milk you would be better off with something like almond milk, rather than cow's milk. But no fruit juice or smoothies.

If you are not drinking enough you may get headaches and become constipated. You can also tell if you are getting dehydrated by looking at your urine, which should be straw-coloured.

Basically, you should be drinking enough fluid so that you are going to the loo to wee at least 6–7 times over a 24-hour period. After a leading academic gave me this tip, I found myself logging whenever I went, and it was always 5–6 times during the day, and once at night.

You might want to use going to the loo as a cue to do some press-ups and squats. Perhaps 10 press-ups and 10 squats after every loo break? That will really add up.

Katie's story

Katie was one of the volunteers for my recent 'Lose a Stone' TV series. When we first met, back in July 2020, she was 34 years old, a teacher and married with two young kids, aged five and seven. When Katie was younger, she was a keen dancer, with no worries about her weight or what she ate. But after she had her children she not only became far less active, but started eating more junk. Not wanting to waste food, she also began eating whatever the kids left on the plate.

She slowly piled on the weight, and when we met, she was 89.8kg (14st 1lb), with a waist size of 102cm, putting her in the 'obese' range. The blood tests we did also revealed that she was prediabetic, with an HBA1c of 43.3, which is very bad news for someone that young.

Katie knew she needed to do something. She also knew that she would not be able to stick to a standard, slow and steady diet. Nevertheless, when she learnt she would be cutting down to just over 800 calories for three weeks, she found that intimidating.

When I first heard it was going to be just over 800 calories a day, I wondered if that was even possible. You think of 800 calories, and you think that's

112

barely one meal. So, one of the first big surprises was realising how much food you can have for 800 calories, if you follow Clare's recipes. I thought that I was going to get really hungry, but that wasn't the case. I was lucky that my husband, who is very interested in food, was hugely supportive and volunteered to join me. So I would cook meals for us, and separate meals for the kids. It worked surprisingly well.

She felt tired for the first few days of the diet, and 'extremely grumpy', but, by Day 4, when her keto sticks began to change colour, her mood lifted and she realised that she actually felt really good.

I found that having the keto sticks was really helpful, and extremely motivating. It made me think, 'Today is a good day, it's a purple colour, so don't go and ruin it by having a snack.'

In just 10 days, Katie lost 4.5kg, and by the end of the 21-day programme she had lost 7.7kg (1st 2lb) and was down to 82.1kg. Although some of that weight loss was water, much of it was fat. She lost an impressive 12cm off her waist and her HBA1c fell from 43.3 mmol/mol (prediabetic) to 33.5 mmol/mol (healthy).

Since then, she has lost a bit more weight and found a healthy pattern of eating that suits her and her family's lifestyle. She and her husband go low carb during the week, but will then eat foods like pasta and pizza at the weekend. She says that for her the secret is that she preps the family meals in advance (still leaning heavily on Clare's recipes, but with larger portions) and resists the temptation to finish off any food that the kids leave on the plate.

I say to myself, 'Is having that fishfinger or pile of pasta the kids have left really worth it? How am I going to feel when I've eaten it?' The answer is 'no' and 'terrible', so these days I just tip it in the bin.

She also has a different approach to the occasional lapses.

I used to be prone to catastrophic thinking. If I had a biscuit, then I would say to myself, 'I might as well finish the whole pack.' Or if I had a bar of chocolate which I hadn't intended to eat, I would feel so bad about it that I would spend the rest of the day eating junk. These days I don't think like that. I see it as a lapse, not an excuse to eat badly.

She allows her kids to have biscuits, but only a few, and she has found brands that they like and she doesn't, so she is rarely tempted to swoop on the biscuit tin. She is back at school, teaching, and takes in a prepared lunch with her. She has told her colleagues and friends why she wants to keep the weight off, so they don't tempt her with sugary snacks. She has also found that telling them has made her more accountable.

I know I would feel bad if, having made this into a big thing, they saw me sneaking in a biscuit.

She doesn't preach, but she has noticed that many of her fellow teachers now bring in healthier snacks.

Your two-week check-in

While you are doing Stage 1, rapid weight loss, I think it is wise to build in a routine in which every two weeks you pause and check in with yourself, just to assess how things are going. Hopefully you will be feeling in control, slimmer, energised, but it's good to check you're not pushing yourself too hard. Diets can be tough even if you are in good health. Ask yourself:

Are you losing weight?
In the first two weeks of Stage 1, you should see the numbers tumbling on your scales. Studies show you can expect to lose up to 4kg (9lb, or over half a stone) in the first two weeks, with some losing more and some losing less. If your weight is not shifting, double-check you are sticking to 800–900 calories and not unconsciously snacking (that stolen chip off your partner's plate, the extra spoon of yoghurt, a handful of crisps – they all add up). By now you should be in ketosis, which will be helping to keep your hunger under control.

Is your appetite under better control?
Because the food you are eating is very low in carbs, but relatively high in fat, protein and fibre (fibre is a carbohydrate, but not digestible by your body), you should

soon stop feeling hungry. Most people report feeling less hungry by the end of Week 1, and you should find you are less bothered by cravings. If you are still feeling hungry, check you are eating enough protein (50–60g per day) and that you are in ketosis.

Do you have bad breath?

Some people start producing the sweet, fruity smell of ketones on their breath. It's a bit like nail polish remover. This is a good sign and shows the diet is working. Brush your teeth regularly and press on!

Are you feeling light-headed?

You might experience mood swings, irritability and dizziness as you adapt to the ketogenic diet, but this will pass. If you are not already taking a supplement, a good multi-vitamin/mineral tablet that contains magnesium, potassium and vitamins B and D can help, as low levels are linked to fatigue. You may simply be dehydrated, so up your water consumption. Remember, you should be drinking enough water to pass six or seven good volumes of urine a day. If you are on blood pressure medication, it could be that you are now over-medicated. Talk to your doctor.

Are you sleeping OK?

If you are struggling to fall asleep or waking up in the night feeling hungry, try eating your main meal a little later in the day. You may also want to increase the amount of veg and protein that you are eating with your evening meal, as there is evidence that protein and fibre help boost deep sleep. Increasing your activity levels can also help, particularly going for a brisk early-morning walk. This resets your internal clock and improves your mood. Mindfulness and breathing techniques can help too (see pages 134–5).

Are you constipated?

A change from your normal diet can cause temporary constipation, but this can be redressed by increasing your water consumption and adding more non-starchy vegetables to your plate at each meal. Berries, chia seeds or flax seeds can help too, or ask your pharmacist about a natural soluble fibre such as Fybogel or Movicol or lactulose, which work by drawing more fluid into the gut, softening the faeces.

Are you coping emotionally?

You may feel more irritable and possibly 'hangry' but that can often be offset by the pleasure of seeing the weight fall off. A prolonged drop in mood might be something to discuss with a professional. But most people, once they have gone into ketosis, report a boost in energy and mood. Intermittent fasting has also been shown to improve mood, as has cutting out junk food and switching to a Mediterranean-style diet.

Are you managing to stick to the diet most of the time?

My hope is your answer is a resounding 'yes!' But if you find yourself having frequent lapses, you may want to consider slowing things down a bit. Try jumping straight to Stage 2.

Veggies and vegans unite!

There's absolutely no reason why you can't do the Fast 800 Keto if you're a pescatarian (no meat, only fish) or a vegetarian. In fact, we've included lots of lovely fish-based and vegetarian recipes in this book, plus a vegetarian meal planner to get you started.

If you are vegan you will have to be clever in your protein choices, as many 'fake meat' products come with hidden carbohydrates which would take you out of ketosis. Even wholesome vegetable sources of protein, such as legumes and pulses, have quite a high carbohydrate content.

Focus on high-protein foods, such as tofu, tempeh, edamame beans and seitan. Adding a big spoonful of nutritional yeast to soups and sauces can help too (51g of protein per 100g). See page 260 for more protein add-ons.

Because protein is so important, we suggest vegans allow themselves to go over 1000 calories if necessary. You will still lose weight, just not quite as fast, and you may not go into ketosis. But that is OK.

An easy and effective way to keep your protein levels up and help you go into ketosis during Stage 1 is by taking a vegan-friendly protein powder and meal replacement shakes (see www.thefast800.com).

What about exercise?

During this first, rapid weight loss stage, many people worry about doing exercise, wondering if it could be dangerous to do so when eating less than 1000 calories a day. The short answer is 'no', because most of us have a large fat store to draw on, so we aren't going to be running out of energy any time soon. Nonetheless, I do suggest that you start gently, as exercise can make you feel more hungry – I will be going into this in more detail in Chapter 7. During the first week, you are also likely to feel quite drained, but as you go deeper into ketosis your energy levels should return.

I would recommend that if you normally exercise regularly you should keep it up throughout this diet. Exercise will push you into ketosis faster, which means you will be increasing its effectiveness.

At a bare minimum, it's a good idea to schedule a brisk walk into your day, every day – even if it's just 10 minutes around the block.

How to transition to Stage 2

Stage 2 is when you start to introduce more calories, as well as TRE (see pages 82–83), if you haven't already done so. During Stage 2, you're still being quite strict about calories and carbs.

When you start Stage 2, I recommend initially following a pattern of 3:4 intermittent fasting, which means sticking to our 800–900 low-carb recipes from Monday to Thursday, then adding in more protein, fats, carbs and even the occasional alcoholic drink (if you like) over the weekend. You will continue to lose weight, but more slowly, as you gradually move towards a more sustainable way of life. When you get close to your goals, you may want to drop a couple of fast days and follow the 5:2 pattern (eating normally five days a week, and sticking to our 800–900 low-carb recipes on two).

Keep on weighing in

During Stages 1 and 2, I recommend you weigh yourself at least once a week. I know opinions vary on this, but research shows that people who keep a close eye on their weight and act swiftly if it starts to rise are much more successful at losing weight and keeping it off.

One thing to bear in mind, when you make the transition, is that your rapid weight loss may stall for a bit. The dreaded plateau. That is mainly because when you start eating more carbs, the glycogen stores in your muscles will refill, and for every extra gram of glycogen you store, you store 3g of water. So your weight will go up, even though you are still burning through your fat stores. As well as weighing yourself you might want to keep an eye on the tape measure, as this is a more reliable measure of fat loss.

If you do reach a plateau or your weight does start to creep up, you might need to reduce the amount of carbs you are eating on your non-fast days, and check you are not unconsciously nibbling at snacks between meals.

Another option is to increase the number of 800–900-calorie days each week. We have found it is best to keep to a regular pattern each week. Changing your fast days week by week tends to mean you will be less likely to stick to them.

Can I have a little tipple?

While you are trying to lose a lot of weight, fast, my advice is that you cut out alcohol completely. During Stage 2 you can go back to some social drinking at the weekends, but alcohol really isn't great for weight loss for the following reasons:

- It seriously weakens your willpower – I find that once I've had a drink my willpower, always weak to begin with, almost entirely disappears.

- It gives you the munchies. When I am drinking I cannot resist crisps.

- It is extremely calorific. One (large) glass of wine is 230 calories, which is the same as a bar of chocolate or a bowl of ice cream – or a whole extra meal.

What if I get invited round to friends?

In an ideal world, any social engagement should fall on one of your non-fast days if you are on Stage 2 of the

Fast 800 Keto plan. If not, you can adjust your week so that this becomes a non-fast day, to take a little pressure off yourself. But actually, even during Stage 1, once you've got properly under way and are feeling the smug satisfaction of seeing your weight beginning to drop, you should be able to cope with the odd lunch or dinner invitation.

Herewith 10 tips on how to manage these:

1. Let your hosts know beforehand that you are following a healthy eating plan, as this should minimise any undue pressure on the day. You might also need to confess to any health concerns to avoid too much 'oh, but you don't need to lose weight' coercion, which can be quite seductive when you're staring at a loaded pavlova.

2. Offer to bring a dish, and pick something from the menus at the back of this book, or a huge (healthy) salad to share.

3. Bring fizzy water to drink.

4. Time your previous meals so you don't arrive hungry.

5. Decline alcohol.

6. Do not touch the nibbles. Not even one crisp. I find that once I start I don't stop. Try to ensure you are never sitting or standing near them. I once did an experiment in which we asked people to watch a TV drama, and critique it afterwards. In fact we

were interested to see who would eat the snacks placed near them, and how much. One contributor ate a large bowl of crisps (around 800 calories) without appearing to notice.

7. Make a healthy selection from the food on offer, basing your meal on protein and green leafy vegetables or salad.

8. Have a well-prepared 'speech' ready for anyone who tries to persuade you that dieting is pointless or that ketogenic diets are unhealthy.

9. If cravings strike, take a moment to run through a quick deep-breathing exercise.

10. Remind yourself, these get-togethers are all about the people, not the food.

How about going out to a restaurant?

Most restaurants are not particularly diet-friendly, so a little forward planning might be called upon.

1. Check the menu online if you can and decide what you plan to order.

2. Get into the habit of asking for extra salad or extra green vegetables in place of potatoes or rice. For me nothing beats a lovely piece of fish with vegetables.

3. Time your other meal or meals that day so that you

are not starving hungry when you go out.

4. Offer to be the designated driver so you have a good excuse not to drink.

5. Ask for tap water for the table and keep drinking throughout the evening.

6. Refuse bread and breadsticks.

7. If everyone is ordering a starter, ask for a simple green salad.

8. If you can't find a healthy meal which ticks all your Fast 800 Keto boxes, order two starters instead.

9. Eat slowly, putting your knife and fork down between every mouthful.

10. Skip dessert.

Curtis's story

When I first met Curtis, in the summer of 2020, he was 30 years old and unhappy in himself. He had recently returned from a teaching job in China and was living with his parents. His beloved grandmother had recently died from Covid and he was comfort-eating. He had put on a lot of weight and was very stressed.

Although he told me he had always been 'the fat kid', he had never been this big before. He weighed in at 95.7kg (just over 15 stone). His BMI, 32.5, put him in the 'obese' category, and I was particularly concerned about his 112cm (44in) waist.

When I measured his blood pressure, it was way too high, and when we tested his bloods his cholesterol and his blood fats were truly shocking for such a young man.

Curtis also had a big neck – 43cm (17in). This extra fat around his windpipe was causing him to snore, very loudly, and I was convinced that if he did nothing about it he was likely to develop sleep apnoea. This is when you stop breathing during the night for up to 20 seconds at a time. It leads to high blood pressure, fragmented sleep, loss of libido and feeling shattered all the time.

Things for Curtis were not looking good, but I was convinced my Fast 800 Keto plan could turn his health around, as long as he was prepared to stick to it.

Thankfully, he was a star pupil. Clare provided him with lots of keto-friendly 800-calorie menus and he really got stuck in. Within four days, he had gone into ketosis and rang me to say, 'I'm smiling because the keto test has changed colour. I am so excited to be in ketosis mode.'

I knew he was faithfully following the diet because every week he'd send me a picture of his latest keto stick.

He decided to try TRE and stick to eating two meals a day: a late breakfast at around 10am, then an early evening meal which he would normally finish by 6pm. This meant that he was eating within an eight-hour window and fasting, overnight, for 16 hours.

In the morning I might have a couple of eggs or some cheese and mushrooms and spinach (the superfood!).

And then in the evening it was chicken or fish and lots of vegetables. The food I missed most was white rice with my curry, but it didn't take long to get me converted to the idea of cauliflower rice, and now I can't imagine eating anything else.

In just three weeks, Curtis lost 11.3kg (1½ stone), and had slimmed down to 84.4kg (just over 13 stone). His blood pressure, blood fats and cholesterol score all fell, returning to normal, healthy levels, and he also stopped snoring. He told me he felt 'fabulous'.

Curtis then decided to move on to Stage 2 of the diet and chose a 3:4 pattern of eating, being strict with himself during the week, and letting go (a little) at the weekends.

He reached his target weight of 74kg (11½ stone) over the next few weeks, having lost a total of 21.7kg (3½ stone) and 25cm (10in) off his waist. I am delighted to say that 18 months later, he has kept all that weight off. So how does he do it?

I am strict with myself from Monday to Thursday, sticking to around 1000–1400 calories per day, eating lots of protein and lots and lots of vegetables. I don't drink alcohol at all during those days. I weigh myself several times a week and, though I typically put on about 1kg over the weekend, I know most of that is fluid and will soon be gone.

I've got used to cooking classic dishes which are healthier and lower in carbohydrates, so I usually carry on doing that over the weekend. But if I get invited out for a meal with friends or there's some sort of celebration going on, then I don't really restrict myself. Equally, I don't go crazy any more. These days I can eat one or two biscuits rather than the whole pack.

If I have a bit of a blow-out (the other day I cooked for a Moroccan-themed party with 12 courses with lots of wine) I'll just fast the next day, sticking to 800 calories and no carbs. It's not hard, I just don't get hungry any more.

As part of his lifestyle change, Curtis has bought a bike and is now cycling as much as possible.

Every week is different, but on average I manage about 40 miles per week. I love it. I am 3½ stone lighter than I was and full of energy. I feel so much better, a lot more confident and with so much more bounce.

Curtis's top tips:

- *Don't worry about a bit of yo-yoing. Over the last 18 months I've put some weight back on (overeating at Christmas and again at Easter), and then lost it again. But now that I'm not bingeing I find it much easier to maintain my weight. In fact, it gets easier because my metabolism has improved and I have been building a bit of muscle as well.*

- *Keep busy. It's when you're sitting watching TV that boredom kicks in and you find yourself thinking about having a snack. When I am at work, teaching, it's relatively easy, because I am on my feet and busy. It is during the holidays, or at weekends, that I am tempted. I know, from long experience, that there are certain points in the day when I will feel hungry, such as 2 o'clock in the afternoon. So, I make sure that I am out cycling or walking or doing something. By 4pm I'm not hungry any more.*

- *Explore and self-experiment until you find a rhythm that works for you.*

Stage 3: the way of life

Well done! Getting this far is a real achievement. You should be feeling healthier, sleeping better, and you will have dropped a few sizes – so this is a good time to buy yourself some new clothes to celebrate. You will have more energy, and many of our dieters report they feel happier, brighter and lighter, more confident and in control.

But you can't go back to your old way of living and eating. You need to be honest with yourself: the reason you gained weight in the first place was because you were eating and/or drinking too much. You need to find an enjoyable way of living which also prevents creeping weight gain.

As you know, the third and final stage of the Fast 800

Keto is based around a Mediterranean-style diet. But what exactly is that? A group of Spanish researchers have come up with a scoring system, which is widely used by international researchers, and which I have adapted. You get a point for every 'yes' answer. A score of 10 is good, but the higher the score the better.[43]

1. Do you use olive oil as your main cooking fat and dressing?

2. Do you eat two or more portions of vegetables a day? (1 serving = 200g/7oz)

3. Do you eat two or more portions of fruit a day?

4. Do you eat less than one serving of processed meat a day? (1 serving = 100g/3.5oz)

5. Do you eat plain yoghurt at least three times a week?

6. Do you eat three or more servings of legumes – e.g. peas, beans, lentils – a week? (1 serving = 150g/5.25oz)

7. Do you eat three or more servings of wholegrains a week? (1 serving = 150g/5.25oz)

8. Do you eat oily fish, prawns or shellfish three or more times a week? (100–150g/3.5–5.25oz)

9. Do you eat sweet treats like cakes, biscuits, etc, less than three times a week?

10. Do you eat a serving of nuts (30g/1oz) three or more times a week?

11. Do you cook with garlic, onions and tomatoes at least three times a week?

12. Do you sit at the table to eat at least twice a day?

13. Do you drink sweet, fizzy beverages less than once a week?

NB:

- Potatoes do not count as a vegetable

- Processed meat includes ham, bacon, sausages and salami

- Wholegrains include quinoa, whole rye and bulgur wheat

- Nuts should include walnuts, almonds and cashew nuts, and should be unsalted

It's good for your mood as well as your waist

There is abundant evidence that the Med diet is a fantastic way of keeping your body and brain in good shape, as well as boosting your mood. In one study, called Smiles, Professor Felice Jacka and her colleagues at the Food and Mood Centre in Melbourne, Australia, showed that switching people from eating a typical Australian diet (high in ultra-processed foods) to eating a Med-style diet led to big improvements in mental health, in just 12 weeks.[44] Surprisingly enough, the researchers also showed it was no more expensive eating healthily than eating badly. Cut out the takeaways and snacks and you will find you are saving money.

One of the things you want to know about any dietary approach is whether people can stick to it, long-term. In a remarkably long study, called DIRECT, researchers in Israel randomly allocated 322 overweight men and women to either a low-fat diet, a low-carb diet (Atkins) or a Mediterranean diet, and then followed them for six years.

Although, initially, the low-carbers lost the most weight, by the end of six years it was those who had been following the Mediterranean diet who came out on top, with an average weight loss of 3.2kg. That figure looks more impressive when you realise that over six years most people put on around 3kg. The Med dieters also saw the biggest improvements in blood fats, blood sugars and insulin levels.[45]

Some general rules to keep you on track

Catch weight regain before it escalates

Down the years I have talked to many weight loss specialists, looking for answers to the fundamental question, how do you keep on track, long-term? The first thing they all say is: don't think you can go away at the end of a diet, any diet, and eat 'normally'. Normally for you is usually too much, that's why you put on weight in the first place. Maintaining awareness and conscious control of how much you're eating is really important.

Second, keep accountable. You can weigh yourself regularly, or put a tape measure around your stomach, or track your blood sugars, whatever it is that works for you. In long-term studies, the people who've lost weight and kept it off are almost always regular self-weighers. It's much easier to catch weight regain before it's gone too far than wait and have a bigger hurdle to jump.

Third, you have to change your environment, so it is easier to stick to your goals. In other words, keep tempting treats out of the house.

Fourth, tell friends and family. Say, 'It's going to be hard. And there will be times when I'm going to fall off the wagon. But I need you there to encourage me.'

Beware snacks and snacking

Contrary to what the food manufacturers claim, 'eating little and often' is NOT a good thing. In fact, studies show that regular snacking (the classic 'five small meals a day') is the best way to put on weight. Compared to 30 years ago, we not only snack more but eat more when it comes to our regular meals. The evidence is that the more we snack the more we eat overall. So do try to avoid them.

That said, if hunger beckons, rather than succumb to the temptation for something starchy and sweet, try and go for something healthy. Here are a few high-protein, low-carb snacks to have at the ready:

• Nuts: a small handful of almonds (10 weigh around 10g) should be enough to take the edge off your appetite. Because of their tough structure and large amounts of fibre, quite a lot of the fat in nuts will not be absorbed by your body. In fact, it has been estimated that 15% of the calories you take in when you eat them goes straight out the other end.

- Hard-boiled egg: one medium-sized egg is 78 calories, contains 7.7g of protein and no carbs.

- Veggie dips: sticks of cucumber, red peppers or broccoli dipped in guacamole make a healthy keto snack. You can buy guacamole in tubs from most supermarkets, or make it yourself by mashing up a ripe avocado with red onion and lime juice. A whole avocado comes in at 300 calories, so you wouldn't want to be eating more than a quarter in one go. But the good news is that it contains lots of fibre, minerals and vitamins, and has hardly any carbs.

Try to reduce stress and improve your sleep
Stress makes successful weight loss harder because stress hormones, such as cortisol, interfere with hunger signalling, making you more likely to be tormented by cravings, and they also instigate metabolic changes that encourage your body to hold onto fat.

Lots of us already have stressful lives and starting on a diet, any diet, can be stressful too. There will be times when you are really busy and up against a deadline, nowhere near a healthy meal and far too close to a convenient but unhealthy snack. There will also be times when you've had bad news, the kids are screaming and all you want is some sugary comfort food. When things get difficult, willpower crumples and you could easily find yourself undoing all your good work.

So, it is a great idea to have a few stress-busting techniques up your sleeve to calm your stress response in heated moments, and hopefully improve your sleep quality too: mindfulness, breathing exercises, maximising your gut health, to name a few. 'Headspace' is one of many apps which will teach you how to meditate and practise mindfulness to reduce anxiety and stress. Do shop around to find a method that works for you.

Also crucial for keeping your cortisol levels regulated and your stress levels down is getting enough sleep. In my book *Fast Asleep*, I offer lots of different tips and techniques to help you sleep better and longer. Often, the simplest ideas work the best. Try this breathing exercise, which is recommended by NHS Choices. I find it really useful for reducing stress and helping me go back to sleep if I've woken in the night. You can do it standing, sitting or lying, but you get the most benefit if you make it part of your daily routine.

- Start by breathing in as deeply as you can, through your nose, without forcing it, to a count of four.

- Hold it for a count of two.

- Then, gently exhale, through your mouth, to a count of four.

- If you keep doing this for a few minutes, you will

find that your heart rate slows down and you will begin to feel calmer.

Dr Gary Lamph's story

Gary is 44 years old, and a senior research fellow in mental health at the University of Central Lancashire. He is also an experienced cognitive behavioural therapist and treats patients who are keen to turn their lives around. He is married to Sharon, a nurse, and has two boys, aged 16 and 19. He told me he had always been a bit of a yo-yo dieter, but during the Covid pandemic he reached 17st 9lb (112kg), with a BMI of 38.7, his heaviest ever. He started on the Fast 800 Keto in early 2021 and in a few months not only lost 4 stone (25kg) but regained his zest for life. I particularly like the way he used his expertise as a mental health specialist to keep on track, developing strategies to overcome common weight loss hurdles. This is his story.

I realised I had to do something about my weight when I was out with my wife on a short walk and I kept having to stop because my legs were so tired. My wife had also noticed that I regularly stopped breathing for periods during the night, which suggested I had a condition called sleep apnoea. So I went to my doctor and discovered that on top of everything else I had high blood pressure, and high cholesterol. My doctor wanted to start me on medication but I asked, 'Is there anything else I can do?' And he said, 'Lifestyle. I will give you six months to turn your life around.'

So Gary decided to do some research, and came across the Fast 800 Keto.

Before starting, I made a list of my problems and identified the goals I wanted to achieve and worked out how I would measure those goals.

One of my goals was I wanted to lose weight because I felt it would make me more confident. So I wrote down, 'On a scale of 0 to 8, where am I now? Where do I want to be? And when?'

There was also the problem of the high blood pressure and cholesterol. I have a family history of heart disease; men in my family have died of heart attacks in their early fifties or even in their forties. So I decided to keep a daily record of my weight change, and to keep track of my blood pressure and cholesterol levels.

I began the day after my 44th birthday, at the end of January 2021. During the first week on the diet I developed keto flu. I felt tired and headachy. The thing that kept me going was knowing what it was that I wanted to change. And knowing that the keto flu would pass. I was also doing it with my wife, and that was a big plus. When there are two of you doing it together, if one of you is having a bad day then the other can pull you through it.

I went into ketosis within five days. I remember seeing the colour change on the keto sticks, and celebrating. I thought that to lose weight I would have to do massive amounts of exercise, so I was surprised that your programme begins with only a modest increase in activity.

One of the first things I noticed, when I went into ketosis, was this huge improvement in energy and also in my cognitive ability. I am a researcher, so my job requires me to be relatively sedentary but I have to do a lot of thinking and writing. Being able to think so clearly was a big plus.

In less than three months he lost nearly 4 stone and 11in (28cm) off his waist.

As the weight started to fall off, I was able to go for much longer walks, and those walks turned into runs. I then fell in love with running. I've never been able to run before because of my weight. By now I was doing twice weekly HIIT exercise as well as running.

I run on an empty stomach and I feel absolutely fine. I can only assume the energy is coming from the fat I'm burning.

Be warned, at some point you will probably plateau. It happened to me after about 10 weeks. Instead of feeling depressed or frustrated, I used this as an opportunity to try something else. What could you do differently? You could increase your time-restricted eating. It might be that you need to cut back on the carbs a bit further for a while. It might be that you need to increase your physical activity. Plateaus are often temporary. My weight began to fall again once I made some subtle changes to my plan.

Gary's tips for how to avoid common mental traps:

I have been a practising cognitive behavioural thera-pist for over 10 years and have experience of working with people with eating problems, including binge eating. Food can be very emotional, both positive and negative. The way you think affects how you react, which affects how you see and feel emotionally and physically. You have to learn to challenge your thinking.

- *A common trap is thinking along the lines of, 'What's the point, my family are eating all this lovely food, why don't I just take the night off?' The problem here is that you are not seeing the bigger picture. What you have to recognise is that it is the 'lovely stuff' they are eating that is responsible for making you overweight and is making you ill. It is the stuff that makes you feel rubbish, keeps your weight up and is making you old before your time.*

- *Another mental trap to be aware of is 'all-or-nothing thinking'. You eat the biscuit and you* think, 'I failed, I might as well eat the rest of the packet.' This is known as self-sabotage. These days, I sometimes sneak across the road and buy a sausage roll, but I don't then eat loads more junk on top of that.

- If you have cravings, try urge surfing. I used to be able to eat takeaways until I felt sick; now I say to myself, 'Gary you've had enough. Have a glass of water. If you sit with the urge for long enough it will pass.'

- I weigh myself every day so I can see the impact of the decisions I've made. Don't wait until the end of the month, when things may have got worse.

- The things that keep me on track are the support of my wife and family, reminding myself of what my goals are, and stamping on weight gain before I drift. I expect setbacks to happen, but I am now better at spotting them and quick to correct them. For me this has become a way of life.

The secrets of naturally slim people

Some people, partly thanks to their genes, find it much easier to maintain a healthy weight, when surrounded by endless temptation, than others.

A typical example of this is my wife, Clare. She is 60 years old, but she is much the same size and shape as when we first met at medical school, 41 years ago. I suspect she could still fit into the clothes she wore then. Despite having had four children she has never put on weight, never dieted and never bothers to weigh herself. The reason she remains slim is not that she has a super-fast metabolism or a particularly strong will but mainly because she, largely unconsciously, has adopted lots of healthy habits which she sticks to without having to think hard about it.

I am completely different, and probably more typical of most people. I ate a lot of junk food when I was a teenager, but that didn't really matter because I was extremely active. In my twenties, I put on weight because I was still eating a lot of calorie-laden snacks, but sleeping badly and spending less time playing sport.

I continued to steadily put on weight through my thirties and forties, until by my mid-fifties I was nearly 90kg, around 15kg heavier than when I first met Clare. It was only when I was told that I had Type 2 diabetes that we realised I had to act. I lost 9kg and that turned my life around.

Since then, I have kept the weight off, but it isn't effortless. My weight goes up and down, though not by much, and I am constantly aware of the need to self-regulate. I have studied Clare closely, and gleaned some interesting insights from her example. These days, I try to copy what she does.

1. Clare very rarely sits for long. She does most of the household chores and almost all of the gardening,

so she burns a lot of calories through everyday activities. Because I do a lot of writing, I spend too much time sitting down. I have bought a stand-up desk, which I use some of the time, and when I am not using it I set an alarm to make sure I get up for a couple of minutes every hour.

2. Clare also fidgets, a lot. She doesn't watch much TV, but when she does she likes to do something else at the same time, like knitting, or asking me annoying questions about the plot. I love TV and would happily gorge on it. I have to ration myself to a couple of hours a day.

3. Like me, Clare does resistance exercises first thing in the morning. Over the years she has increased the number of push-ups she can do from a couple to around 20. I can still beat her, but that is mainly because I am male and have the genetic advantage.

4. We go for a walk every day, often more than once. When we walk, Clare likes to walk fast, something like 110 steps a minute (which is not far short of jogging). If I am walking by myself I have a tendency to dawdle, but I find listening to music, with a fast tempo, helps push me along.

5. We both cycle into town, when we can. We live at the top of a very steep hill, so it is really hard work on the way home.

6. Clare almost never snacks. She tells me that she likes the feeling of being slightly hungry, the antici-

pation of the meal ahead. I find snacking very hard to resist, particularly when I am bored or stressed. I used to snack on chocolate or biscuits, but these days make do with a small handful of nuts because there are no unhealthy snacks in the house.

7. Clare very rarely eats anywhere but at the kitchen table. I would happily eat in front of the TV, despite the fact that I know it is a really bad habit. Studies have shown that if you eat while watching TV you eat more.

8. Clare has a savoury tooth and she is not particularly interested in sweet things. I love chocolate and if there is any in the house I will sniff it out and eat it up. There is some evidence that sweet or savoury preferences have a genetic component, but be warned, you can put on just as much weight eating savoury snacks as you can eating the sweet stuff.

9. Clare loves vegetables and will fill at least half her plate with them. I have slowly learnt to love vegetables, but even now I am not as generous with the veg as I could be when I am doing the cooking.

10. Clare has taught me to enjoy and savour food. I used to wolf it down, without paying much attention to what I was eating. But, as we have seen, if you eat fast, you eat more. It was striking in Dr Hall's study (see pages 43–45) that when people ate ultra-processed food they ate much faster.

11. When Clare was growing up she occasionally had

puddings, but it wasn't a big deal. Whereas I always expected pudding, which I thought was the best part of the meal. Even now I crave something sweet at the end of a meal, but will usually stick to a bit of fruit or some yoghurt and berries. One rule I have found relatively easy to stick to is that I never order dessert when we go out for meals (but might eat some of Clare's).

12. When we go out for a coffee, Clare sometimes buys a muffin, but rarely feels the need to finish it. I can't do that. If I buy a muffin, or a bit of cake, I will peck away until it is mysteriously gone.

13. When Clare gets stressed, she will go for a walk. When I get stressed, I feel an intense urge (which I normally resist) to go and buy a packet of biscuits.

14. A couple of years ago, we agreed to stick to a 3:4 pattern when it comes to alcohol. We don't drink on Monday to Thursday, only on Fridays and at weekends, and even then, not that much.

15. Clare never weighs herself. She doesn't need to. Her brain somehow just keeps her on track. I weigh myself once a week, as well as occasionally checking my blood pressure and blood sugars. I also wear a tight belt. If I didn't do that, I know that I would put on weight.

Summary

By now you should be ready to put theory into practice. Yes, the first couple of weeks on the Fast 800 Keto can be tough but you will love our recipes and if you stay strong you will achieve your goals. Here are the key points to take on board:

- Accept that you are going to be making some pretty big changes to your life, but they are absolutely worth it.

- Kicking off with rapid weight loss will keep you motivated and will also help preserve your metabolic rate, which will make it easier to keep weight off long-term.

- By cutting back on ultra-processed food and switching to a Mediterranean-style diet, you will be improving not only your body and brain but also your mood.

- Do make sure that you are eating plenty of good-quality protein. Think meat, fish, eggs, tofu, Greek yoghurt, lentils and chickpeas. 15–20% of your diet should be protein, which means that after Stage 1 you should be consuming around 70–100g of protein a day, which is well above the recommended amount of 45g–55g.

- Make sure you are also consuming plenty of fibre, as this will act as a brake on your appetite, as well as feeding the 'good' bacteria in your gut.

- Once Stage 1 is over, you can eat more carbs, but try to stick to complex carbs, like beans and brown rice. Keep away from the processed carbs you find in cakes, biscuits, pies and white bread, as they will send your blood sugar levels soaring and set you up with hard-to-resist cravings.

- Try serving yourself smaller portions than you used to before you embarked on the Fast 800 Keto, and eat slowly and mindfully. Don't be afraid to leave food on the plate.

- Give TRE a go, and if it works for you, stick to it. You should aim to eat within a 12-hour window, maybe even 14:10 (i.e. 14 hours of fasting).

- Weigh yourself regularly – one large study found that people who weighed themselves daily were, on average, 6.5kg lighter at the end of the two-year trial than those who weighed themselves monthly.

- Stay active – this is something that most successful long-term dieters do. The good news is that when people lose weight, they find that activities like walking or cycling become easier and much more enjoyable.

- Cook more – that way you know what is going into the food you're eating. Plus it keeps you on your feet.

- Drink plenty of water and aim for seven wees a day.

- Prioritise sleep – poor-quality sleep raises your stress hormone levels, which leads to increased hunger and cravings, particularly for high-carb foods.

- Limit your alcohol intake – you might even try giving up alcohol completely. But if, like me, you find life is enhanced by a glass of red wine, or a cold beer on a sunny day, then perhaps try a 3:4 rule, where you only drink at weekends, or on special occasions.

- Like Gary, when you are tempted to give up, think about why you've been doing this. You might not adhere to the Kate Moss edict that 'nothing tastes as good as skinny feels', but you want to live to a healthy old age, don't you? You want to be free from disease, fit and happy, able to bend down and to do up your own shoelaces. Whatever your motives were when you started on this plan, it's good to remind yourself of them from time to time.

Cautions & Exclusions

If you have Type 2 diabetes, are on insulin or high blood pressure medication, please talk to your health professional before starting this diet.

*The Fast 800 Keto programme is **not** recommended for people who are underweight and/or experiencing an eating disorder or have a history of eating disorder; children (under 18 years old); Type 1 diabetics; pregnant women; breastfeeding mothers or anyone undergoing fertility treatment; people who have a significant psychiatric disorder; anyone who has moderate or severe retinopathy, epilepsy or gallstones, or who has a significant medical condition or is under active investigation or treatment. For more information, please refer to thefast800.com/frequently-asked-questions/*

7

Exercising and keto

Exercise can and should be included as part of the Fast 800 Keto programme, but it is best if you start off gently. During the first week of the new diet, you are likely to feel drained as your body goes into ketosis, switching from burning sugar to burning fat; then, when you've flipped the metabolic switch, you should feel a real surge in energy, and that is what I want you to really capitalise on.

As we saw in Chapter 3, exercise alone is unlikely to lead to weight loss (that's what the studies show, I'm afraid), but it's absolutely vital in so many other ways: being active and fit means better health and better mood; it can cut your risk of heart disease and stroke by up to 35%, of Type 2 diabetes by up to 50% and of early death by up to 30%.

And don't be daunted by what you might think is involved in getting fitter: the really brilliant thing is that you can quickly and safely overhaul your fitness while doing the Fast 800 Keto, and you don't have to join a gym or pound the pavements to do it.

Get your steps up

As you will see from Wayne's story later in this chapter, if you are not particularly fit, walking is a great place to start. It is a cheap and safe way to exercise and the best time to do it, if you can fit it into your life, is first thing in the morning, before breakfast. That way you not only manage to wake yourself up but you also get exposed to early-morning light. Bright light in the morning helps reset your internal clock, which in turn will help you sleep better at night. If you can't do it then, find another time that works. And it doesn't have to be done in one chunk. Lots of people find it easier to schedule in three brisk 10-minute walks a day. You can find a free app called Active 10 that will guide you at www.nhs.uk/oneyou/active10/home.

HIIT

The idea behind High-Intensity Interval Training (HIIT) is that you really push yourself by doing quick, but intense bursts of exercise, followed by short recovery periods. You shouldn't do HIIT every day and, as with any exercise, if you suffer from underlying conditions seek medical advice first. But it is a really effective way of improving your aerobic fitness in a remarkably short period of time.

HIIT breaks down glycogen, the form in which sugar is stored in your muscles and liver, which means you will go into ketosis faster. This also sets off a cascade of other reactions, including the release of something called 'signalling molecules', which help to stimulate the growth of muscle, including heart muscle.

HIIT is also very effective at targeting visceral fat, burning away the fatty deposits that can lead to insulin resistance and Type 2 diabetes.

Recent studies have shown that as well as improving fitness, HIIT can actually reverse the effects of ageing on mitochondria – the power-houses of our cells. As we age, the ability of mitochondria to obtain energy by burning glucose declines. In tests, however, HIIT boosted the performance of mitochondria by 49% in people aged 18–30, and by a stunning 69% in people aged 65–80.

The other great thing about HIIT is that it's adaptable to your own fitness level and suitable for all ages. So provided you push yourself during each short burst, you should reap the benefits.

The secret to doing HIIT is not speed, but effort. You have to push yourself, whether you're on an exercise bike, doing sprints, jumping jacks or even running up the stairs. As long as you are putting in your maximum effort, at whatever speed that happens to be, it will improve your health. It is about getting your heart rate up during a 20-second burst of activity.

One of the problems with exercise is that it has a tendency to trigger compensatory eating. People go on a treadmill for 30 minutes, burn 300 calories, then reward themselves with a muffin. HIIT seems to be more effective at suppressing your appetite, so this is less likely to happen.

There are lots of different ways to do HIIT. If you have an exercise bike, try the regime I describe below. You can also swap cycling for running up stairs for 20 seconds or putting in short, flat-out sprints when jogging. You can also do it while swimming. Again, it is just a 20-second burst.

If you have an exercise bike at home, try this:

1. Warm up with some gentle cycling.

2. After a minute or so begin pedalling fast, then swiftly crank up the resistance.

3. The level of resistance you select will depend on your strength and fitness. It should be high enough that, after 15 seconds of sprinting, your thighs begin to feel it and your muscles begin to fatigue.

4. If, after 15 seconds, you can keep going at the same pace, the resistance you've chosen isn't high enough. It mustn't, however, be so high that you grind to a halt. It's a matter of experimenting. You'll find that as you get fitter, the level of resistance you can cope with increases. Each 20-second workout should involve maximum effort.

5. After your first burst of fast sprinting, drop the resistance and do three minutes of gentle pedalling.

6. Then do the 20-second sprint again.

7. Finish with a couple of minutes of gentle cycling to

allow your heart rate and blood pressure to return to normal before stepping off the bike.

Resistance training

As well as looking after your heart and lungs through HIIT and regular walking, you need to pay attention to your muscles. Unless you do resistance exercises, you will lose around 3–5% of your muscle mass every decade after the age of 30. And if you are not eating enough protein, the problem is even worse. The best way to counteract this is by maintaining a protein intake of around 70–100g a day and doing regular sessions of strength or resistance training. Not only will this keep you strong and protect you from injury, but it will improve your insulin sensitivity, reducing your risk of Type 2 diabetes.

I am a particular fan of something called High-Intensity Circuit Training (HICT), which involves no equipment, apart from a chair, and which is a mix of resistance training and an aerobic workout. You can do this in just seven minutes and, despite the scary-sounding name, you can make it as intense (or not) as you like. Essentially, you do 12 different exercises, which work different muscles in your body, and you do each one for just 30 seconds, with a 10-second break in between.

Most mornings I get out of bed, activate my 7-minute workout app (there are lots of '7-minute workout' apps you can find online – the J&J version, which I use, is free), and do a series of jumping jacks, wall sits, push-ups, squats, abdominal crunches, triceps dips and the plank – in roughly that order.

The J&J version is the original '7-minute workout' and was developed by Chris Jordan, Director of Exercise Physiology at the Johnson & Johnson Human Performance Institute in Orlando, Florida. He once called it a 'hotelroom workout' because it was designed for people who didn't have the time or equipment to exercise while travelling.

HICT is popular because it is very short, and because it gives one set of muscles a chance to recover while you are working out another set. You start with the upper body, then move on to the lower body. I suggest you start by doing one set of 7-minute workouts three times a week, and if you are super-keen, pick it up from there. There are also excellent exercise programmes on thefast800.com for all levels of fitness.

The best exercise 'cocktail'

The recommended advice – that we all do 150 minutes of moderate-intensity exercise per week – is simple and clear, but the latest science shows that doing a mixture of different exercises is best.

Fascinating data from six studies, which included more than 130,000 adults in the UK, US and Sweden, used mathematical modelling to determine how different combinations of activities – including moderate-to-vigorous exercise (such as brisk walking, running or other activities that increase heart rate), light physical activity (such as housework or casual walking) and sedentary behaviour – affect mortality.[46]

If you are largely sedentary, punctuating your day with 'light activity' is key. According to the researchers, the ideal exercise cocktail consists of 12 minutes of light activity or three minutes of moderate-to-vigorous activity for every hour you spend sitting. You can do this in a chunk, or break it up, but do try to get up and move around every hour. This could be enough to reduce your risk of early death by 30%.

If you've got young children, or an active job which requires you to be on your feet for much of the day, your 'light activity' is covered, and your challenge is merely to find time to squeeze in some proper exercise regularly. But if you work long hours behind a desk, or if you've got into the habit of sitting all day playing computer games or watching TV, a little light activity could save your life.

Even something as fleeting as a four-second burst of exercise has been shown to be worth it. You just need to be active – you could do some squats, a short wall sit, nip out for a brisk walk, or pump out a few jumping jacks.[47]

One way in which short bursts of activity help to optimise health is by waking the body up out of 'sleep' mode, flicking on the digestive switch and making us better able to process nutrients.

Similar research has shown that a 20-second exercise

'snack' (in this case racing up three flights of stairs three times a day for three days a week) is enough to increase aerobic fitness by 5% in six weeks. It also boosts muscle strength and leg power.[48]

10 ways to introduce more activity into your life

1. Buy a bike and cycle when you can. It saves lots of time and money.

2. If your destination is less than a mile away, why not walk? It will take you less time than waiting for a bus or finding somewhere to park.

3. Stand while talking on the phone. You'll burn calories and sound more assertive.

4. Use a basket at the shops rather than a shopping trolley. That way you do a bit of resistance training at the same time.

5. Drink lots of water. This not only keeps you hydrated but also increases the need for bathroom breaks, which means in turn more short, brisk walks.

6. Try, where possible, to take the stairs. I always run up escalators.

7. If you normally take a bus or train to work, get off at an earlier stop than usual and walk the rest of the way.

8. If you drive to work or the supermarket, park at the far end of the car park.

9. Keep resistance bands – stretchy cords or tubes that offer resistance when you pull on them – or small hand weights near your desk. Do arm curls between meetings or tasks.

10. Organise a lunchtime walking group. You might be surrounded by people who are just dying to lace up their trainers. Enjoy the camaraderie and offer encouragement to one another when you feel like giving up.

Wayne's story

I first met Wayne in early 2021 when he volunteered to take part in a TV series I was making called 'The 21-Day Body Turnaround'. Wayne, who is married with three children, was 42 years old, and struggling. His catering business had been hammered by Covid; he was tired, stressed and very overweight. He was desperate to change. Before starting, we carried out a range of tests on him, which revealed he had high blood pressure, high cholesterol and the aerobic fitness of an average 58-year-old. When I gave him the bad news he was visibly shaken.

I knew I was in a bad shape but not as bad as you found. I went to my car after you told me my results and cried. It was a combination of shock and fear. I have a family history of heart disease so I couldn't believe that I'd allowed myself to get to that point.

Wayne decided he wanted to go straight onto the Fast 800 Keto. He started using the recipes that Clare had provided and embraced TRE from the get-go. His oldest son, Jack, and his partner, Jen, joined him.

They were hugely supportive. They weren't as strict as me, they did more like 1000 calories and I know my son had the occasional cheeky takeaway because I would find the remains in the bin. But he was good enough not to eat them in front of me.

I asked Wayne not only to change what he ate but to try and increase his average step count. I also suggested he join in some online HIIT classes, which started quite gently but then built up over the course of the three weeks we were filming the series.

At the start I was doing only about 4000 steps a day, but I soon built that up to 10,000 steps. I would look at my monitor, see where I was, and when the kids had gone to bed I would go out for a walk with the dog and get in lots of extra steps. It was pretty challenging because normally at this time of the day I would sit down in front of the TV with a snack and a drink.

I warned Wayne that the first few days on the Fast 800 Keto would be tough. And they were.

I didn't really feel hungry, but I felt incredibly lethargic. Doing the exercises was really hard. Then suddenly it was like a switch had gone off, I got a lot more energy and the exercises became far easier. Almost addictive. My son did the workouts with me and he would often join me for the walks so we would chat and that was lovely. Time together which we wouldn't have had if I was slumped in front of the TV.

He was amazed by how quickly everything improved.

I think the change in my mood was the biggest thing that I noticed first. I rediscovered a taste for life. If my kids wanted to play then I was there to play.

By day 10 I had already lost 4.5kg (10lb) and my skin was clearer, I felt better, I looked better. I didn't look bloated and I was really astonished by how quickly that all happened.

In just three weeks Wayne lost 8kg (18lb) and 8cm (3in) off his waist. His blood pressure came down, his stress levels improved (we measured his cortisol levels) and he went from having the aerobic fitness of a 58-year-old to that of a 44-year-old (just over his real age).

Since then he has stuck to his new regime, continuing to lose weight and get fitter.

I eat a lot more protein, particularly fish. Far more than I have ever had before in my life. We also eat far more veg than we ever did and less starchy foods like potatoes or rice. I still eat junk food some-times. I am human. But we are much stricter with the kids, and give them fruit to eat rather than biscuits or a cake as a snack. It's amazing how quickly they change.

My family was really proud of me. My partner and son both noticed the impact on their bodies and brains of eating differently, eating right rather than eating junk.

The biggest thing I would say is focus on being what you want to be. I didn't want to be the guy I was before. But if you do slip up, well, that's fine, just put it behind you and get straight back on it.

My current regime is that I do a regular 20-minute HIIT workout twice a week and do lots of walking. It is about seeing what you can fit into your life. I have also started cycling again with my dad, which is lovely. I don't panic about doing exercise: if it fits in it fits in. If it doesn't it doesn't.

And finally...

I do hope you have success with this diet, which is based on the work of numerous scientists from around the world, far too many to mention individually, though I would like to say a special thanks to Prof Roy Taylor, Prof Mike Lean, Prof Susan Jebb, Prof Stephen Simpson and Dr Mark Mattson.

Remember, you don't have to lose a lot of weight to see big improvements in health. Indeed, even just changing your eating habits, cutting out ultra-processed foods and cooking more meals from scratch will make a huge difference to how you look and feel. Obviously, I hope you will do this. But there is also a wider message that needs to be delivered loud and clear to our politicians. While we can, individually, decide to do something about weight gain by reducing our reliance on factory-made food, it is imperative that governments also introduce legislation to curb the food giants.

That, in the end, was what made a difference when it came to curbing the power of the big cigarette companies.

According to a recent study by the Institute of Health Metrics and Evaluation, published in the *Lancet*, unhealthy diets are now responsible for 11 million preventable deaths every year – more deaths than from smoking.[49] This is not to mention the hundreds of billions of dollars spent treating complications of obesity and Type 2 diabetes.

Most governments have favoured a hands-off voluntary arrangement with food manufacturers, encouraging them to make their products healthier. In reality, this has made very little difference. A study by researchers from Oxford University, which looked at foods sold in English supermarkets between 2015 and 2018, found they were selling less sugar-laden fizzy drinks, the direct result of a sugar tax introduced in 2018, but there was no evidence that anything else had improved.

We know, from the long war on tobacco, what works and what doesn't. Expecting food manufacturers to police themselves doesn't work. Repeatedly telling people these foods are bad for them might make a small difference, but probably won't.[50]

The only way to make a big difference is to tax unhealthy foods, subsidise healthier alternatives and reduce or ban advertising of junk food, particularly to kids. Despite numerous reports, which have said much the same thing, governments are often reluctant to act due to fears of being accused of implementing a Nanny State. That has to change, and soon.

Recipes

by Dr Clare Bailey
and food writer Kathryn Bruton

Our recipes are specially designed to help you through Stage 1 of the Fast 800 Keto programme. You may find it easier to use our meal plans at first, to ensure that you are getting the right daily amounts of protein and carbs, while keeping to the 800–900 calorie count. But do also feel free to put your own menus together, mixing and matching different recipes to suit. Just keep an eye on the nutritional information to ensure you are meeting the Rule of 50 – that is, less than 50g carbs and at least 50g protein per day (see pages 80-81).

A few things to note:

- When it comes to non-starchy veg, no calorie counting is required. So pile your plate high with greens and salad, and add any of the veg sides on pages 242-49 for free.

- On hungry days you can go to 1000 cals – choose from the list of protein add-ons on pages 258–61 to supplement any of the recipes.

- Dressings need to be considered, but if they encourage you to eat more nutritious veg we regard this as a good thing, so be aware of the extra calories but don't get too hung up on them! See our simple dressing recipes on pages 250–51, all of which are less than 100 cals per portion.

When you move on to Stages 2 and 3, do keep using our recipes as a base repertoire. They are all designed to be easily adapted – either by doubling up portion sizes or adding in extra foods. We have included 'non-fast day' tips and options at the end of most of the recipes to help you do this. But get creative: stick to a lowish-carb Med-style way of eating and you can't go wrong. Just remember to keep an eye on your protein intake – which by now should be around 70–100g per day, i.e. almost twice what you ate on Stage 1.

Bon appétit!

You can follow Clare on Instagram @drclarebailey for tips and more recipes

BREAKFAST

Breakfast Traybake

Per serving: 361kcals, 25g protein, 4.5g carbs

Take the fuss out of making a full cooked breakfast! While the oven works its magic, you can get on with your morning. Simple swaps, such as vegetarian sausages and halloumi, will make this a nutritious meat-free meal.

Serves 2
Prep time: 5 minutes
Cook time: 25 minutes

- 1 large tomato, sliced into 4
- 2 portobello mushrooms
- 2 Cumberland or vegetarian sausages, halved lengthwise
- 2 rashers back bacon (or 100g block halloumi, sliced in 2)
- 1 tbsp olive oil
- 2 medium eggs

1. Preheat the oven to 200°C/fan 180°C/gas 6 and line a baking sheet with non-stick baking paper.

2. Place the tomato, mushrooms, sausages and bacon (or halloumi) on the prepared tray. Drizzle the

olive oil over the tomato and mushrooms and season them with salt and freshly ground black pepper. Place in the oven and bake for 20 minutes.

3. Remove from the oven, break the eggs onto the tray and bake for another 5 minutes, or until the yolks are just set.

NON FAST-DAY: Serve with a thin slice of wholegrain or seeded sourdough buttered toast.

Keto Pancakes with Yoghurt and Berries

Per serving: 187kcals, 8g protein, 4.5g carbs

Super-easy to make, these pancakes are delicious served with yoghurt and berries.

Serves 4 (makes 12 small pancakes)
Prep time: 5 minutes
Cook time: 8 minutes

   30g ground almonds
   60g cream cheese
   2 medium eggs
   ½ tsp vanilla extract (or lemon zest)
   15g butter
   200g fresh berries, such as strawberries, raspberries
      or blueberries
   4 tbsp full-fat Greek yoghurt

1. Whisk together the ground almonds, cream cheese, eggs and vanilla extract in a medium bowl until smooth.

2. Melt half the butter in a large non-stick frying pan over a medium heat. Drop in 4 tablespoons of batter to make 4 small pancakes. Cook for about 2 minutes, or until golden, then flip and cook on the other side for the same amount of time. Transfer to a plate and continue with the rest of the butter and batter.

3. Serve the pancakes topped with fruit and yoghurt.

TIP: Any leftover pancakes can be frozen for another day.

NON-FAST DAY: Top the pancakes with a handful of flaked almonds or pecans, or an extra handful of berries.

Rapid Bircher with Apple and Cinnamon

Per serving: 300kcals, 8g protein, 16g carbs

This scrumptious take on a Bircher muesli is ready in seconds but can also be made in advance and kept in the fridge for a ready-made breakfast.

Serves 2
Prep time: 5 minutes

1 tbsp chia seeds
2 tbsp rolled oats
170g full-fat Greek yoghurt or non-dairy equivalent
1 red apple, such as Gala, coarsely grated
30g pecans, roughly chopped
½ tsp ground cinnamon

1. Place all the ingredients in a bowl with a pinch of salt and 2–3 tablespoons of water and mix well.

2. Eat immediately or leave in the fridge for up to 24 hours (see tip below).

   TIP: The chia seeds will thicken with time, so simply add 1–2 tablespoons of water to loosen the mixture.

   NON-FAST DAY: Increase the portion size and add extra pecans.

Scrambled Eggs with Smoked Salmon, Feta and Avocado

Per serving: 320kcals, 19g protein, 2g carbs

Scrambled eggs are my favourite breakfast, especially with the addition of smoked salmon. This is a particularly filling version that will power you well into the day. Add a pinch of dried chilli flakes to give it a kick, or scatter some freshly chopped herbs, such as parsley or dill, over the top before serving.

Serves 2
Prep time: 3–5 minutes
Cook time: 3–4 minutes

> 4 medium eggs
> 10g butter or 1 tsp olive oil
> 60g smoked salmon, diced
> 40g feta, crumbled
> ½ large avocado, peeled, destoned, sliced and dressed with a little fresh lemon juice
> 2 tsp mixed seeds (around 10g)

1. Whisk the eggs in a bowl and season with salt and freshly ground black pepper.

2. Melt the butter in a non-stick saucepan over a low heat. Pour in the eggs and stir continually for 3–4 minutes, or until creamy and just starting to set.

3. Immediately remove from the heat and stir in the

salmon and feta. Season with a generous grind of black pepper.

4. Serve with the sliced avocado alongside and the mixed seeds scattered all over.

NON-FAST DAY: Serve with a thin slice of wholegrain buttered toast and add marmite for extra flavour, if you like.

Baked Eggs with Spinach and Chorizo

Per serving: 361kcals, 29g protein, 0.5g carbs

A fantastic high-protein breakfast that will kick-start your day. It would also make an appetising lunch or supper with a mixed salad (see dressings on pages 250–51).

Serves 2
Prep time: 5 minutes
Cook time: 12–15 minutes

300g frozen spinach, defrosted
1 tsp olive oil
50g good-quality chorizo, diced
25g Cheddar, coarsely grated
4 medium eggs

1. Place the spinach in a sieve and press out any excess liquid.

2. Heat the oil in a non-stick frying pan or casserole with a lid and fry the chorizo over a medium heat for 2–3 minutes, or until crisp. Add the spinach and Cheddar and stir to combine. Season with salt and ground black pepper.

3. Make four small holes in the mixture and break an egg into each one. Cover the pan with a lid (or a large piece of foil) and cook gently over a low heat for 4–5 minutes, or until the whites are set but the yolks are still runny. Serve immediately.

TIP: For a quick hit of extra heat, garnish with some chilli flakes.

NON-FAST DAY: Serve with a thin slice of wholegrain or sourdough toast. A nice addition – mix ½ teaspoon paprika with 2 tablespoons of Greek or natural yoghurt and spoon this over the dish before serving.

Cheese and Chive Muffins

Per serving: 194kcals, 10g protein, 1.5g carbs

These cheesy muffins make a tasty alternative to the starchy toast we often crave in the morning. They are quick to make and will keep in the fridge for a day or two in an airtight container. They benefit from a few seconds in the microwave before eating to bring out the flavours. Try them with wilted spinach on the side.

Makes 6 muffins
Prep time: 5–7 minutes
Cook time: 15 minutes

115g ground almonds
½ tsp bicarbonate of soda
2 medium eggs
50ml milk
1 tsp fresh lemon juice
50g Cheddar, grated
5–10g fresh chives or parsley, finely chopped
25g pine nuts

1. Preheat the oven to 200°C/fan 180°C/gas 6 and line a muffin tray with 6 muffin cases.

2. Mix the ground almonds and bicarbonate of soda in a large bowl with a generous pinch of salt and plenty of ground black pepper, making sure everything is evenly combined.

3. Add the remaining ingredients and mix well.

4. Spoon the mixture into the muffin cases and bake for 15 minutes, or until golden and risen.

TIP: Keep any uneaten muffins in the freezer. They can be defrosted easily, ready for a quick breakfast on the go.

NON-FAST DAY: Serve two muffins per person, instead of one, and enjoy with a colourful dressed salad.

Microwave Eggs with Spinach and Mackerel

Per serving: 299kcals, 20g protein, 0.5g carbs

This high-protein breakfast makes a great start to the day. Keep a close eye when cooking eggs in the microwave. If left for too long they can explode!

Serves 1
Prep time: 2–3 minutes
Cook time: 4–5 minutes

   50g frozen spinach
   1 tbsp crème fraîche
   50g cooked smoked mackerel, skin removed and broken into pieces
   1 medium egg

1. Place the spinach in a ramekin and microwave for 3 minutes. Stir in the crème fraîche and mackerel, and season with salt and ground black pepper.

2. Crack the egg on top and use a sharp knife to pierce three holes in the yolk.

3. Cook in the microwave for 1 minute 30 seconds, checking every 15 seconds from then on, until the white is set and the yolk is still runny (or cooked to your liking).

TIPS: Use a standard 9 or 10cm ramekin for this recipe. Smoked salmon can be used in place of mackerel.

Cashew, Vanilla and Fig Breakfast Shake

Per serving: 183kcals, 10g protein, 12g carbs

A smooth, luxurious shake with a delicate flavour.

Serves 2
Prep time: 2 minutes

150g silken tofu
100ml full-fat cow's milk
25g cashews
1 dried fig
1 tbsp vanilla extract
¼ tsp ground cinnamon (optional)

1. Place all the ingredients in a blender and blitz until completely smooth.

TIP: If this is one of your main meals, serve as a single portion. The shake will keep in the fridge for up to 24 hours. You can use almond milk instead of cow's milk, in which case calories per serving will be 157 and protein 8g.

NON-FAST DAY: Increase or double the portion size.

BRUNCH & LUNCH

Pea and Mint Soup

Per serving: 161kcals, 8g protein, 9g carbs

The classic combination of pea and mint tastes wonderful in this easy-to-make soup. Served hot or cold, it makes an ideal packed lunch – just pour it into a flask or jar. Swirl in a tablespoon of full-fat yoghurt to make it extra creamy, or scatter over a tablespoon of toasted seeds for a bit of crunch.

Serves 2
Prep time: 2–3 minutes
Cook time: 8–10 minutes

> 1 tsp olive oil
> 30g smoked lardons or pancetta cubes
> 200g frozen peas
> 300ml hot chicken or vegetable stock (made with ½ stock cube)
> 50ml full-fat milk
> 4 sprigs of fresh mint, leaves picked (or ½ tsp dried mint)

1. Heat the oil in a medium saucepan and fry the lardons for 3–4 minutes (2–3 minutes if using pancetta).

2. Add the peas and stock, bring to the boil and simmer for no more than 5 minutes.

3. Remove from the heat, add the milk and mint and blitz with a stick blender until smooth. Season with salt and plenty of ground black pepper.

TIP: Adjust calories if using non-dairy milk (50ml full-fat dairy milk = 34 cals)

NON-FAST DAY: Serve with a wholegrain bread roll and/or top with some grated Cheddar or more fried smoked lardons or pancetta.

Chunky Courgette and Dill Soup with Prawns

Per serving: 162kcals, 17g protein, 5g carbs

When a soup has texture to it, it feels more filling and satisfying. Leftover chicken would work well in place of prawns. This is also a great way to use up a summer glut of courgettes.

Serves 2
Prep time: 5 minutes
Cook time: 10 minutes

> 1 tbsp olive oil
> 1 medium leek, trimmed, quartered lengthwise and sliced
> 2 medium courgettes, trimmed, quartered lengthwise and sliced into cubes
> ¼ tsp dried chilli flakes
> 600ml hot chicken or vegetable stock (made with 1 stock cube)
> 10g fresh dill (or parsley)
> 150g cooked prawns

1. Place the oil in a saucepan over a medium heat and sauté the leek and courgettes for 4 minutes, adding a splash of water if necessary.

2. Add the chilli flakes and stock, then cover with a lid and simmer for 5 minutes.

3. Transfer half the soup to a blender, add the dill

(or parsley) and blitz until smooth. Return to the saucepan and remove from the heat.

4. Stir in the prawns so that they warm but don't cook any more. Season to taste and serve immediately.

TIPS: Raw prawns can be used instead of frozen; simply add to the soup and simmer for an extra 2–3 minutes, or until they have turned pink. A squeeze of lime juice adds extra zing. To prepare this soup ahead, complete to the end of Step 3, then store in the fridge until ready to serve. Warm it up and add the prawns immediately before eating.

NON-FAST DAY: Serve with a thin slice of sourdough toast or a wholegrain bread roll.

Curried Smoked Haddock Chowder

Per serving: 281kcals, 34.5g protein, 10g carbs

This light and aromatic soup makes a remarkably indulgent low-calorie meal.

Serves 2
Prep time: 7–10 minutes
Cook time: 15–20 minutes

> 2 smoked haddock fillets (around 300g total weight)
> 200ml full-fat milk
> 1 tbsp olive oil
> 1 medium leek, halved and sliced
> 1 medium carrot, trimmed and diced
> ½ tbsp mild curry powder
> 1 tsp ground turmeric (optional)
> 1 tbsp chopped fresh parsley

1. Place the fish in a small saucepan, cover with the milk and gently heat. Once the milk starts to bubble, remove from the hob, cover with a lid and set aside.

2. Place the olive oil in another saucepan and sauté the leek and carrot over a medium heat for about 5 minutes, or until softened. Add a splash of water if they begin to stick.

3. Add the curry powder, turmeric, if using, and 350ml water. Bring to the boil, simmer for 10 minutes, then remove from the heat.

4. Remove the skin from the fish and flake the flesh into the vegetable mixture. Stir the poaching milk into the pan and season with salt and ground black pepper. Garnish with the chopped parsley to serve.

TIPS: It is worth keeping a few fillets of haddock in your freezer – the remaining ingredients in this soup are likely to be in your cupboard or fridge. Onions can be used instead of leeks, and you can play around with adding different greens, such as spinach, green beans and finely sliced cabbage.

NON-FAST DAY: Serve the chowder with a poached egg on top and/or add 2–3 tablespoons of cooked pearl barley to the chowder in Step 4.

Goat's Cheese Frittata with Greens and Diced Figs

Per serving: 301kcals, 21g protein, 10g carbs

We love our eggs – they are low carb, high protein and incredibly nutritious. When our children are home, this makes an easy breakfast or brunch and keeps us full for ages. The goat's cheese adds a salty tangy flavour, which is balanced by the sweetness of the fig. Parmesan or Cheddar would work, too. Serve warm with a mixed salad (see pages 250–51 for dressings) or let it cool and cut it into slices for a delicious packed lunch.

Serves 4
Prep time: 7 minutes
Cook time: 10–12 minutes

> 1 tbsp olive oil or small knob of butter
> 1 medium onion, peeled and diced
> 60g leftover leafy green veg (cooked weight)
> 8 medium eggs, lightly whisked
> 80g goat's cheese, sliced
> 3 dried figs, diced

1. Place the oil or butter in a large non-stick frying pan over a medium heat and sauté the onion for 4–5 minutes, or until soft and translucent. Meanwhile, preheat the grill to high.

2. Add the greens to the frying pan and heat through.

Stir in the eggs, half of the goat's cheese and all the figs. Season generously with salt and freshly ground black pepper. Cook over a medium heat for 2 minutes, using a wooden spoon to draw the egg towards the middle of the pan and allowing it to run back towards the side of the pan as it cooks.

3. While the egg is still slightly runny, top with the remaining slices of cheese and place the pan under the grill with the handle away from the heat. Cook for about 4 minutes, or until the top is set and slightly browned.

NON-FAST DAY: Increase the portion size and/or add roasted squash in Step 2.

Protein Wrap Two Ways

Per serving: 192kcals, 16g protein, 3.5g carbs

So simple to make, these are brilliant lunchbox fillers – and a healthy alternative to a starchy wrap. Best eaten the same day.

Serves 1
Prep time: 2–3 minutes
Cook time: 4 minutes

    2 medium eggs
    1 tsp wholemeal flour
    ½ tsp olive oil or butter

1. Crack the eggs into a cup or small bowl and whisk lightly.

2. Add the flour, a pinch of salt and freshly ground pepper and whisk again until smooth, making sure there aren't any lumps.

3. Place the olive oil or butter in a medium non-stick frying pan and use a piece of kitchen roll to spread it evenly over the base.

4. Pour in the egg mixture and cook gently over a medium heat for 2 minutes. Flip the wrap over and cook for 1 minute more. Remove from the pan and leave to cool before filling with one of the combinations overleaf.

Beetroot, Rocket and Feta

Per serving: 279kcals, 21g protein, 10g carbs

Prep time: 5 minutes

>   1 cooked beetroot, sliced into matchsticks
>   Small handful of rocket
>   20g feta

1. Place the beetroot on one half of the wrap and top with rocket and crumbled feta. Season with salt and ground black pepper, roll up and serve.

Smoked Salmon, Cream Cheese and Capers

Per serving: 379kcals, 29g protein, 8g carbs

Prep time: 5 minutes

>   2 tbsp cream cheese
>   50g smoked salmon
>   1 tsp capers
>   A few Little Gem or romaine lettuce leaves

1. Carefully spread the cream cheese over the wrap. Top with the salmon, capers and lettuce. Season, roll up and serve.

   TIP: Rocket or other lettuce leaves would work well, too.

Spinach and Ham Omelette

Per serving: 148kcals, 13g protein, 0g carbs

We often have this tasty omelette for brunch. Serve tangy sauerkraut or kimchi on the side for a spicy kick (no calorie counting needed) and your microbiome will love it, too. Definitely a family favourite.

Serves 2
Prep time: 2–3 minutes
Cook time: 4–5 minutes

> 30g baby spinach, roughly chopped
> 2 slices smoked ham, diced
> ½ tbsp olive oil
> 4 medium eggs
> 10g Parmesan, grated

1. Place the oil in a small-medium-sized non-stick frying pan over a medium heat. Add the spinach and ham and fry for about 2 minutes, or until the spinach has wilted.

2. Meanwhile, crack the eggs into a small bowl, season with a little salt and some freshly ground black pepper and whisk lightly. Pour the eggs into the pan and, using a wooden spoon or spatula, draw in the egg from the edge of the pan to allow it to run back towards the side of the pan as it cooks.

3. When the eggs are almost set, scatter the cheese on

top, then fold the omelette in half and remove it from the pan.

NON-FAST DAY: Increase the portion size and/or serve with a dressed salad sprinkled with toasted nuts or seeds.

Protein Salad with Tuna, Roasted Red Peppers, Edamame and Harissa

Per serving: 436kcals, 27g protein, 11.5g carbs

This satisfying salad is packed with protein and vibrant flavours, enhanced by the unusual harissa dressing. The Little Gem leaves act as healthy taco shells but you could add extra leaves to the filling or serve them on the side, too, if you like.

Serves 2
Prep time: 10 minutes

1 × 145g can tuna in oil, drained
60g pitted black kalamata olives, halved
100g roasted red peppers, sliced
100g frozen edamame beans, defrosted
2 Little Gem lettuces, torn into leaves
20g mixed seeds

Dressing
2 tbsp harissa
2 tbsp olive oil
80g silken tofu
2 tbsp cider vinegar

1. To make the dressing, place all the ingredients in a blender and blitz until completely smooth. Season with salt and freshly ground black pepper.

2. In a separate bowl, mix together the tuna, black olives, roasted peppers and edamame beans. Add

the dressing and toss to coat.

3. Arrange the leaves on two plates and spoon some mixture into each one. Top with the seeds and serve.

TIP: To prevent any tofu going to waste, simply make a larger quantity of the dressing and keep it in the fridge for another day. It will keep for up to five days. Served as a dip with crudités, it would make a quick, healthy snack.

NON-FAST DAY: Increase or double the portion size and/or add 2–3 tablespoons of cooked quinoa, bulgur wheat or brown rice.

Waldorf Salad

Per serving: 417kcals, 32g protein, 7g carbs

Forget those unsatisfying diet salads, this is a gratifying and filling meal– with texture and crunch in the apples and walnuts and quality protein in the chicken.

Serves 2
Prep time: 10 minutes

>   100g rocket or mixed leaves
>   1 red apple, cored, finely sliced and tossed with a
>   little fresh lemon juice
>   1 large celery sick, diced
>   200g cooked skinless chicken, diced
>   6–8 radishes, trimmed and sliced
>   40g walnuts, roughly chopped
>   30g soft blue cheese, such as Roquefort,
>   crumbled

Dressing
2 tbsp full-fat Greek yoghurt
1 tbsp good-quality full-fat mayonnaise
Zest and juice of ½ lemon

1. To make the dressing, mix all the ingredients together and season with salt and freshly ground black pepper.

2. In a separate bowl, combine the rocket or mixed leaves, apple, celery, chicken and radishes. Pour in

the dressing and toss to coat well. Top with the walnuts and blue cheese to serve.

NON-FAST DAY: Serve with a thin slice of sourdough toast, a wholegrain bread roll and/or 2–3 tablespoons of cooked quinoa or bulgur wheat.

Cheesy Asparagus Prosciutto Bites

Per serving: 116kcals, 9g protein, 0.8g carbs

These savoury wraps can be eaten straight from the pan, or on the go. A colourful salad with a light dressing (see page 250) would go well with them.

Serves 2
Prep time: 5 minutes
Cook time: 5 minutes

> 4 slices prosciutto ham
> 4 asparagus spears, woody ends broken off
> 20g Gruyère cheese (or Jarlsberg), sliced into 4
>   equal lengths
> ½ tbsp olive oil

1. Lay the slices of prosciutto on a clean, flat surface. Chop each piece of asparagus in half and lay two pieces in the middle of each slice of ham.

2. Place a piece of cheese on top of the asparagus and roll the ham up tightly and securely.

3. Place a frying pan over a medium heat, add the oil and fry the rolls for 2–3 minutes, turning them to make sure each side is nice and crispy.

4. Remove from the pan and place on a piece of kitchen roll to absorb any excess oil. Leave to cool or serve warm.

Lunchbox Salad of Broccoli, Feta and Piquanté Peppers

Per serving: 320kcals, 14g protein, 11g carbs

The sweet and mildly spiced peppers are a perfect foil for the tangy feta in this simple salad. Get to love your broccoli, if you don't already, for its taste and versatility, as well as its long list of health benefits, which include being low in calories but high in the nutrients, vitamins and antioxidants that help to reduce the risk of cardiovascular disease, Type 2 diabetes, inflammation and cancer – it really is an impressive 'superfood'!

Serves 1
Prep time: 5–7 minutes
Cook time: 1 minute

½ small head of broccoli, cut into bite-size florets
4 piquanté red peppers from a jar, quartered
25g feta, crumbled
10g pumpkin seeds
1 tbsp olive oil
½ tbsp cider vinegar

1. Place the broccoli in a saucepan of salted boiling water and simmer for 1 minute. Drain immediately and refresh under cold water.

2. Place the peppers, feta and pumpkin seeds, along with the cooked broccoli, in a bowl (or lunchbox)

194

and drizzle the oil and vinegar all over. Toss to coat and season with salt and freshly ground black pepper.

TIP: Piquanté peppers are readily found in supermarkets, but you can use roasted red peppers from a jar instead.

NON-FAST DAY: Increase or double the portion size and/or serve with 2–3 tablespoons of cooked brown rice, quinoa or wholewheat pasta.

Cheesy Biscuits with Two Delicious Dips

Per serving: 100kcals, 6g protein, 1g carbs

These biscuits make a great snack on their own, or a dunking device for the dips. They will keep for up to a week in an airtight container.

Makes 10 biscuits
Prep time: 8–10 minutes
Cook time: 15 minutes

> 60g Cheddar, coarsely grated
> 60g Parmesan, finely grated
> 60g ground almonds
> 3 tbsp mixed seeds
> 1 medium egg white

1. Preheat the oven to 190°C/fan 170°C/gas 5 and line a large baking sheet with non-stick baking paper.

2. Place all the ingredients in a bowl, season generously with freshly ground black pepper and mix together well.

3. Use a dessert spoon to scoop the mixture onto the prepared sheet, pressing each biscuit flat with the back of the spoon. Place in the oven and bake until golden – about 15 minutes.

4. Remove from the oven and leave to cool on a wire rack.

Beetroot and Blue Cheese

Per serving: 189kcals, 7g protein, 3g carbs

Serves 2
Prep time: 5 minutes

> 1 medium cooked beetroot
> 2 tbsp full-fat Greek yoghurt
> 25g blue cheese, such as Stilton
> 30g walnuts, chopped

1. Place all the ingredients in a bowl with a generous pinch of salt and freshly ground black pepper. Blitz with a stick blender until smooth.

Smoked Mackerel and Lemon

Per serving: 165kcals, 12g protein, 0.5g carbs

Fresh herbs, such as dill or parsley, or finely chopped rocket or spinach, would make a lovely addition to this dip.

Serves 2
Prep time: 5 minutes

> 100g cooked smoked mackerel, skin removed
> 2 tbsp full-fat Greek yoghurt
> Zest of 1 lemon

1. Mash the mackerel fillets in a bowl with a fork until broken down but still a bit chunky.

2. Mix in the yoghurt and lemon zest, and season with freshly ground black pepper.

NON-FAST DAY: Increase the portion size or serve the dips with fingers of toasted wholemeal pitta or thin wholegrain crackers.

TIP: These dips would also work beautifully with fresh vegetable crudités, such as celery, radish, cucumber, peppers and crispy Little Gem lettuce leaves.

Roasted Broccoli and Kale with Halloumi and Harissa

Per serving: 396kcals, 18g protein, 9.5g carbs

Nothing quite beats the ease of a traybake. This one is packed with flavour. A real winner.

Serves 2
Prep time: 5 minutes
Cook time: 20 minutes

> 200g tenderstem broccoli, woody stems trimmed
> 50g kale, tough stalks removed
> 2 tbsp cider vinegar
> 1 tbsp olive oil
> 120g halloumi, cut into thin slices
> 10g pine nuts or mixed seeds
> 2 tbsp full-fat Greek yoghurt
> 1½ tbsp harissa paste

1. Preheat the oven to 200°C/fan 180°C/gas 6 and line a baking sheet with non-stick baking paper.

2. Place the broccoli and kale in a bowl and toss with the vinegar, olive oil and a generous pinch of salt and freshly ground black pepper, making sure everything is thoroughly coated.

3. Spread the vegetables over the prepared baking sheet. Lay the halloumi on top and bake in the oven for 15 minutes.

4. Remove from the oven, scatter over the pine nuts

and cook for a further 3–5 minutes, or until the pine nuts are nicely browned.

5. Remove the baking sheet from the oven and set aside. Beat the yoghurt and harissa together, then pour the mixture over the traybake and toss everything together.

NON-FAST DAY: Increase the portion size and/or serve with 2–3 tablespoons of cooked brown rice or a mixture of wild rice and brown basmati.

Simple Saag with Tandoori Halloumi

Per serving: 516kcals, 24g protein, 20g carbs

The halloumi adds texture and protein to this flavoursome vegetarian curry. For extra protein, drizzle with a spoon of Raita (see page 251) or Greek yoghurt, or top it with a poached egg.

Serves 2
Prep time: 5 minutes
Cook time: 15 minutes

- 2 tbsp olive oil
- 1 medium onion, peeled and finely chopped
- 2 garlic cloves, peeled and finely chopped
- 2.5cm piece of fresh root ginger, peeled and finely chopped
- 260g frozen spinach
- 1 × 400g can chopped tomatoes
- 1½ tbsp tandoori curry powder
- 125g halloumi, cut into 2cm cubes
- 30g cashews

1. Using 1 tbsp olive oil, sauté the onion, garlic and ginger in a large frying pan over a gentle heat for 2–3 minutes.

2. Add the spinach, tomatoes and 1 tablespoon of the curry powder and bring to a simmer. Cook for 8 minutes, stirring from time to time to break up the blocks of spinach. Season with salt and freshly

ground black pepper, transfer to a bowl and keep warm.

3. Wipe the pan clean and return to the heat. Fry the halloumi in the remaining olive oil for about 3 minutes, or until browned and crisp. Stir in the remaining curry powder and cook for 30 seconds more.

4. Spoon the spinach mixture into bowls and top with the halloumi and cashew nuts.

TIPS: The tandoori halloumi makes a great quick snack. The spinach mixture could be made ahead or doubled up and kept in the fridge for a few days.

NON-FAST DAY: Increase the portion size and serve with 2–3 tablespoons of cooked brown rice or a wholemeal chapati. You could also stir in some extra protein, such as edamame beans or cooked chicken.

Tomato, Chorizo and Mozzarella Pizza with Rocket

Dough per serving: 313kcals, 9.6g protein, 12g carbs

Topping per serving: 160kcals, 12g protein, 2g carbs

There is something indulgent about a pizza, but the standard base is starchy and fattening. This dough – which uses protein-rich almonds instead of white flour – is much lighter. We suggest a tomato, chorizo, mozzarella and rocket topping, which is our family favourite, but you can be creative with your own variations.

Makes 5 pizza bases/Topping for 1
Prep time: 15 minutes
Cook time: 15 minutes

> 140g ground almonds
> 60g psyllium husk
> 2 tsp baking powder
> 1 tsp fine sea salt
> 3 egg whites
> 200ml warm water
> 50ml olive oil
> 2 tsp cider vinegar
>
> *For the topping:*
> 1 tbsp tomato purée
> 15g chorizo, diced
> ¼ ball mozzarella, torn

½ tsp dried oregano
Small handful of rocket

1. Preheat the oven to 200°C/fan 180°C/gas 6.

2. Mix all the dry ingredients together in a bowl. Add the egg whites, warm water, olive oil and cider vinegar and give it all a quick mix until well combined. It should form a dough-like ball.

3. With a few drops of olive oil on your hands to prevent sticking, divide the mixture into 5 balls. Place one ball on a piece of non-stick baking paper and place another piece of baking paper on top. Press down with your hands, then use a rolling pin to roll out the base until it is just 1–2mm thick. Repeat with the remaining balls or store them in the fridge or freezer for another day.

4. Transfer the non-stick baking paper to a baking sheet. Spread with the tomato purée, then scatter the chorizo and mozzarella over the top. Sprinkle with the oregano and season with a little salt and plenty of freshly ground black pepper. Bake in the hot oven for about 15 minutes, or until it is just getting crispy and golden brown around the edges.

5. As soon as it comes out of the oven, scatter with the rocket to serve. You can add extra leafy salad to fill half the plate to get your greens – no counting required – and see page 250 for a light dressing.

TIP: If you have calories to spare or are feeling you need a few extra, you can add ½ tbsp grated Parmesan.

NON-FAST DAY: Use the dough to make four pizzas instead of five.

MAINS

Tomato and Pepper Sauce Three Ways

Per serving: 540kcals, 12.5g protein, 57g carbs

This versatile tomato and pepper sauce makes a great base for all sorts of savoury meals. We use it as a base for steamed fish, baked meatballs and a soup with chicken and spinach (see pages 208-11). The recipe below makes one batch, but you could double up the ingredients and use half now and store half in the freezer for another day.

Makes 1 batch
Prep time: 10 minutes
Cook time: 20 minutes

> 2 medium red onions, peeled and finely chopped
> 2 garlic cloves, peeled and finely chopped
> 2 tbsp olive oil
> 3 peppers, any colour, deseeded and cut into
>   2cm pieces
> 1 × 400g can chopped tomatoes
> 2 tsp paprika
> ½ tsp dried chilli flakes (optional)

1. Place a frying pan over a medium heat and sauté the onions and garlic in the oil for 3–4 minutes, or until softened.

2. Add the peppers, tomatoes, paprika, chilli flakes (if using) and 100ml water and stir to combine. Cover with a lid and simmer for 15 minutes, stirring half-way through. Season with salt and freshly ground black pepper.

Steamed Fish with Tomato and Pepper Sauce

Per serving: 434kcals, 28g protein, 29.5g carbs

The tomato and pepper sauce marries beautifully with white fish. Add half a plate of green veg to make a light meal with fabulous Mediterranean flavours.

Serves 2
Prep time: 3 minutes
Cook time: 25 minutes

  1 × batch Tomato and Pepper Sauce (see page 206)
  1 tbsp green or black olives
  70g green beans, trimmed
  2 × 120g thick, skinless white fish fillets (such as cod or haddock)
  1 tbsp olive oil
  2 lemon wedges, to serve (optional)

1. Preheat the oven to 200°C/fan 180°C/gas 6.

2. Cut out two large rectangles of non-stick baking paper and place half the Tomato and Pepper Sauce in the centre of each. Top with the olives, green beans and fish, then drizzle the olive oil over. Season with salt and freshly ground black pepper.

3. Fold the baking paper over and carefully seal all the edges to make parcels. Place on a baking sheet and bake in the oven for 25 minutes.

4. Serve with a wedge of lemon if using.

   NON-FAST DAY: Increase or double the portion size and/
   or roast small cubes of butternut squash alongside the
   fish and serve with 2–3 tablespoons of cooked green
   lentils.

Baked Meatballs with Mozzarella

Per serving: 459kcals, 25g protein, 14.5g carbs

Serve these meatballs with a very generous helping of greens or thin beans. A hit of chilli works well here, too.

Serves 4
Prep time: 3 minutes
Cook time: 20 minutes

- 1 × batch Tomato and Pepper Sauce (see page 206)
- 12 small, good-quality beef, pork or lamb meatballs (around 350g)
- 125g mozzarella, torn into pieces

1. Preheat the oven to 200°C/fan 180°C/gas 6.

2. Pour the Tomato and Pepper Sauce into a baking dish and place the meatballs on top. Scatter the mozzarella pieces over and season with salt, freshly ground black pepper and a pinch of chilli flakes if you like. Place in the centre of the oven and bake for 20 minutes.

TIP: Fresh basil leaves make a delicious garnish for this dish.

NON-FAST DAY: Increase the portion size and/or serve with wholegrain noodles or 2–3 tablespoons of cooked brown rice.

Easy Chicken, Spinach and Tomato Soup

Per serving: 393kcals, 24.5g protein, 28.5g carbs

This is a hearty, chunky soup that will be ready in minutes and leave you feeling full and satisfied.

Serves 2
Prep time: 2–3 minutes
Cook time: 5–6 minutes

> 1 × batch Tomato and Pepper Sauce (see page 206)
> 1 chicken or vegetable stock cube
> 100g frozen spinach
> 120g cooked chicken, diced

1. Place the Tomato and Pepper Sauce in a medium saucepan and stir in the stock cube, spinach and 450ml water. Bring to the boil, then reduce the heat and simmer for 5 minutes, or until the spinach has fully defrosted.

2. Add the chicken and simmer for 30 seconds more to heat through. Season with salt and freshly ground black pepper.

   NON-FAST DAY: Increase the portion size and serve with a thin slice of wholegrain or seeded sourdough bread.

Baked White Fish with a Parmesan Crust

Per serving: 249kcals, 28g protein, 0.7g carbs

Forget fattening battered or breaded fish that piles on the pounds and try this crispy oven-baked version instead. Even reluctant fish eaters will love it!

Serves 2
Prep time: 10 minutes
Cook time: 15 minutes

> 1 tbsp olive oil
> 20g ground almonds
> 2 x 120g skinless white fish fillets
> 20g Parmesan, finely grated
> ¼ tsp paprika

1. Preheat the oven to 200°C/fan 180°C/gas 6 and line a baking sheet with non-stick baking paper.

2. Pour the olive oil into a bowl. Place the ground almonds in a separate bowl and add a generous pinch of salt and freshly ground black pepper.

3. Dip the fish in the oil to coat all sides, then dip it in the ground almonds. Transfer to the prepared baking sheet and bake in the oven for 5 minutes.

4. Meanwhile, mix the Parmesan and paprika together in another bowl. After 5 minutes, remove the sheet from the oven and sprinkle the Parmesan all over the fish. Return to the oven to bake for

another 10 minutes, or until it is nicely browned. (You may need to cook the fish for a few minutes longer if the fillets are thick.)

5. Serve with plenty of cooked green veg or a crunchy salad.

TIP: Using defrosted frozen fish is fine.

NON-FAST DAY: Increase or double the portion size and/or serve with 2–3 tablespoons of cooked quinoa or lentils.

Cauliflower Rice Risotto with Chicken, Edamame and Roasted Red Peppers

Per serving: 355kcals, 25g protein, 11.5g carbs

Here, cauliflower rice takes the place of traditional risotto rice. The chia seeds give the risotto a smooth, creamy texture, while keeping starchy calories to a minimum. Serve with half a plate of green veg, a salad or some baked courgettes (see page 242).

Serves 4
Prep time: 15 minutes
Cook time: 15 minutes

- ½ medium cauliflower, cut into small florets and leaves roughly chopped
- 2 tbsp olive oil
- 1 medium onion, peeled and finely chopped
- 2 garlic cloves, peeled and finely chopped
- 1 tbsp chia seeds
- 1 vegetable or chicken stock cube
- 100g frozen edamame beans, defrosted
- 100g roasted red peppers (from a jar), finely chopped
- 200g cooked chicken, finely sliced
- 60ml full-fat crème fraîche
- 50g Parmesan, finely grated

1. To make the cauli rice, place the cauliflower in a food processor and blitz until fine. If your food

processor is small, do this in two batches (or grate by hand).

2. Place the oil in a large frying pan and sauté the onion for 3–4 minutes, or until it starts to brown. Add the garlic and cook for 1 minute more. Stir in the cauli rice, 400ml water and the chia seeds, and crumble in the stock cube.

3. Bring to the boil, then reduce the heat and simmer, stirring from time to time, for 7–10 minutes, until the liquid has almost completely evaporated and the cauliflower is cooked but still retains a little bite.

4. Stir in the edamame beans, roasted red peppers, chicken, crème fraîche and Parmesan. When thoroughly mixed and heated through, remove from the heat and season with salt and freshly ground black pepper.

TIP: The base of this risotto will lend itself to any flavours or toppings. Some diced fried chorizo and leftover leafy greens would work well, as would lots of lightly fried mushrooms. For alternative proteins, try prawns, halloumi or bacon, or see pages 258-60.

NON-FAST DAY: Increase or double the portion size, add 1–2 tablespoons of cooked quinoa to the pan in Step 4 and/or replace 100ml of water with white wine in Step 2.

Beef Stroganoff

Per serving: 493kcals, 27g protein, 3.5g carbs

Who says diets are about deprivation? This rich and
indulgent dish is full of flavour and will leave you
feeling pleasantly satiated. It's delicious served with
cabbage pappardelle (see page 243), steamed greens,
or cauliflower mash (see page 246).

Serves 2
Prep time: 8–10 minutes
Cook time: 10-12 minutes

    2 tbsp olive oil
    1 medium onion, peeled and thinly sliced
    300g chestnut mushrooms, sliced
    1 garlic clove, peeled and finely chopped
    1 sirloin steak (around 225g), excess fat removed and
        thinly sliced into 1cm strips
    80ml full-fat crème fraîche
    ½ tsp paprika
    1 tbsp English mustard

1. Heat 1 tablespoon of the olive oil in a medium non-
   stick frying pan and fry the onion and mushrooms
   for 8–10 minutes, until softened and browned.
   Add the garlic and fry for a further minute. Use a
   slotted spoon to transfer the mixture to a bowl.

2. Place the remaining oil in the pan and, when hot,

add the steak and fry it for 1½ minutes, stirring it once or twice while cooking. Cook for 30 seconds more if you like your meat well done.

3. Return the onion and mushrooms to the pan and stir in the crème fraîche, paprika and mustard – it will bubble immediately. Remove from the heat and season with salt and freshly ground black pepper.

NON-FAST DAY: Increase the portion size and serve with 2–3 tablespoons of cooked brown rice.

Black Bean Chilli

Per serving: 172kcals, 8g protein, 16g carbs

This tasty dish provides plenty of gut-friendly fibre to keep your microbiome healthy and happy. Serve with steamed greens, such as sliced savoy cabbage or cavolo nero, and a side of cauli rice (see page 245).

Serves 4
Prep time: 10 minutes
Cook time: 20 minutes

  2 tbsp olive oil
  1 medium onion, peeled and finely chopped
  1 red pepper, deseeded and finely chopped
  150g mushrooms, finely chopped
  1 tsp ground cumin
  2 garlic cloves, peeled and finely chopped
  1 tsp chilli flakes
  1 × 400g can black beans, drained
  1 × 400g can chopped tomatoes
  1 vegetable or chicken stock cube
  4 tbsp full-fat yoghurt
  1 tbsp chopped fresh coriander or parsley to
    serve (optional)

1. Place the olive oil in a saucepan over a medium heat. Add the onion, pepper and mushrooms and sauté for 3–4 minutes, or until softened.

2. Add the cumin, garlic and chilli flakes and cook for a further 30 seconds.

3. Mash half of the beans roughly, then add them to the pan, along with the whole beans. Stir in the tomatoes and stock cube and simmer for 15 minutes.

4. Season with salt and freshly ground black pepper and serve topped with a generous spoonful of yoghurt and the herbs scattered over (if using).

TIP: If you have any leftovers, use them to make another dish. Thinly slice one aubergine and fry it in a couple of tablespoons of olive oil. Layer the slices in a small baking dish with the leftover chilli and top with 30g grated Cheddar. Bake in an oven preheated to 200°C/fan 180°C/gas 6 for 20–25 minutes, or until the cheese is golden and bubbling.

NON-FAST DAY: Increase or double the portion size and serve with 2–3 tablespoons of cooked brown rice.

Pulled Pork with Cider Vinegar

Per serving: 387kcals, 32.7g protein, 8g carbs

Traditionally slow-cooked over wood, this simple, oven-baked version is succulent and tender and has a lovely smoky flavour.

Serves 6
Prep time: 7–10 minutes
Cook time: 4.5 hours

- 1 boned and rolled pork shoulder joint (roughly 1kg)
- 2 medium onions, peeled and roughly chopped
- 150ml cider vinegar
- 2 tsp smoked paprika
- 2 bay leaves or ½ tsp cloves
- 1 tbsp honey

1. Preheat the oven to 140°C/fan 120°C/gas 1.

2. Place the pork in a medium casserole with a lid. Add the onions, cider vinegar, 1 teaspoon of the smoked paprika and the bay leaves or cloves, and pour in enough water to half cover the pork. Put on the lid and place in the oven for 3.5–4 hours, depending on the size of the joint, basting occasionally.

3. Carefully remove from the oven, scatter the remaining paprika over the pork and drizzle with the honey. Return to the oven, uncovered, increase

heat to 190°C/fan 170°C/gas 5 and cook for 30 minutes.

4. Take the casserole out of the oven and carefully lift the pork onto a tray. Remove any excess fat and use two forks to shred the meat. Discard the bay leaves or cloves from the sauce, return the shredded meat to the casserole, stir everything together and season with salt and freshly ground black pepper.

5. Serve with a salad.

TIP: Choose a fatty joint of pork.

NON-FAST DAY: Roast small cubes of butternut squash on a baking tray alongside the pork in Step 3.

Speedy One-Pan Thai Red Curry with Salmon

Per serving: 401kcals, 26g protein, 7g carbs

A fragrant, creamy keto curry, which is super-easy to make. Add extra tenderstem broccoli, if you wish.

Serves 4
Prep time: 8 minutes
Cook time: 10–12 minutes

> 1 tbsp olive oil
> 1 red (or white) onion, peeled and roughly chopped
> 5cm piece of fresh root ginger, peeled and chopped
> 2 tbsp Thai red curry paste
> ½ × 400ml can full-fat coconut milk
> 200g tenderstem broccoli
> 4 salmon fillets (around 450g total weight)

1. Heat the oil in a deep frying pan and sauté the onion and ginger, stirring often, until softened – about 3 minutes.

2. Add the curry paste and coconut milk and bring to the boil. Season with salt (or ½–1 tablespoon of fish sauce, if you have it) and freshly ground black pepper.

3. Place the broccoli on top of the sauce, followed by the fish. Cover with a lid or a piece of foil and simmer over a medium heat for 8 minutes.

4. Serve with Cauli Rice (see page 245) or Cabbage Pappardelle (see page 243).

TIPS: A squeeze of lime or lemon juice before serving will make all the flavours sing. Thai curry pastes differ in flavour and intensity – start with 2 tablespoons and add more if necessary. The jar may tell you how much paste is needed per 400ml can of coconut milk. Stir the coconut milk well before pouring it into the pan as it often separates in the can. You can also buy 200ml pouches, ideal for this recipe.

NON-FAST DAY: Serve with wholegrain noodles or 2–3 tablespoons of cooked brown rice.

Tarragon Chicken with Bacon and Mushrooms

Per serving: 355kcals, 32g protein, 1g carbs

This classic dish is one of our favourite comfort foods and, like many of these recipes, works well for the whole family. So, on a fast day, Michael will have a portion served with cooked greens, a salad, cauli rice or steamed cabbage pappardelle (see pages 245 and 243), while we add a few tablespoons of wholegrains, such as quinoa or brown rice.

Serves 2
Prep time: 5–7 minutes
Cook time: 30–35 minutes

   2 chicken thighs, bone in, skin on and trimmed
   1 tbsp olive oil
   2 rashers smoked back bacon, diced
   150g chestnut or white mushrooms, sliced
   1 garlic clove, peeled and finely chopped
   1 tsp dried tarragon
   3 tbsp crème fraîche
   1 tbsp cider vinegar

1. Preheat the oven to 200°C/fan 180°C/gas 6.

2. Season the skin of the chicken with salt and freshly ground black pepper, drizzle over half the olive oil and roast in the oven for 30–35 minutes, or until the juices run clear when pierced with a knife.

3. Meanwhile, heat the remaining oil in a frying pan and fry the bacon and mushrooms for 2–3 minutes, or until lightly browned. Add the garlic and tarragon and fry for 1 minute more.

4. Just before the chicken is ready, remove the frying pan from the heat and stir through the crème fraîche and vinegar. Season to taste with salt and freshly ground black pepper.

5. Serve the sauce with the chicken on top and plenty of steamed greens.

NON-FAST DAY: Increase or double the portion size and/or roast small cubes of butternut squash alongside the chicken in Step 2, or serve with 2–3 tablespoons of cooked puy lentils.

Quick Veg and Salmon Stir-Fry with Ginger and Oyster Sauce

Per serving: 355kcals, 21g protein, 9g carbs

Using a shop-bought stir-fry mix and cooked salmon, this recipe requires little-to-no effort and beats any takeaway.

Serves 2
Prep time: 3–4 minutes
Cook time: 4–5 minutes

> 2 tbsp olive oil
> 1 garlic clove, peeled and sliced (optional)
> 5cm piece of fresh root ginger, peeled and finely chopped
> 1 × 300g pack stir-fry vegetables
> 1 tbsp soy sauce
> 1 tbsp oyster sauce
> 2 fillets cooked salmon (about 180g total weight), roughly broken into chunks
> ¼–½ tsp dried chilli flakes

1. Heat the olive oil in a wok or a deep frying pan. When sizzling hot, stir-fry the garlic and ginger for 30 seconds, then add the vegetables and stir-fry for 2–3 minutes.

2. Add the soy and oyster sauces and cook for 30 seconds more to heat through.

3. Finally, stir through the salmon, season and

sprinkle with chilli flakes to serve.

NON-FAST DAY: Increase or double the portion size and/or serve with wholegrain noodles or 2–3 tablespoons of cooked brown rice.

Aubergine Parmigiana with Lentils

Per serving: 322kcals, 14g protein, 10g carbs

Aubergine Parmigiana is comfort food at its finest.
Serve with a generous colourful salad.

Serves 4
Prep time: 10 minutes
Cook time: 50–55 minutes

> 5 tbsp olive oil
> 3 garlic cloves, peeled and roughly chopped
> 1 × 400g can chopped tomatoes
> 1 beef or vegetable stock cube
> 2 small aubergines, trimmed and sliced lengthwise
>   into 0.5cm strips
> 125g tinned green lentils
> ½ tsp dried oregano
> 1 × 125g ball of mozzarella, thinly sliced
> 40–50g Parmesan, finely grated

1. Preheat the oven to 200°C/fan 180°C/gas 6.

2. To make the tomato sauce, place 1 tablespoon of
   the olive oil in a saucepan over a medium heat and
   fry the garlic for about 1 minute, or until just starting to brown. Stir in the tomatoes and stock cube,
   and simmer for 3–4 minutes. Remove from the
   heat and blitz with a stick blender until completely
   smooth. Season with freshly ground black pepper.

3. Place a large frying pan over a high heat and add 1

tablespoon of the olive oil. Lay half the aubergines in the pan and fry for 3–4 minutes, or until nicely browned. Flip over, add another tablespoon of olive oil and cook on the other side for the same amount of time. Repeat with the remaining aubergines and oil – you should only need to cook in two batches.

4. To assemble the Parmigiana, pour the lentils into the base of a medium baking dish. Layer half the aubergines on top and season generously with salt and freshly ground black pepper. Top with half the tomato sauce, half the oregano and half the mozzarella. Repeat with the remaining aubergines, sauce, mozzarella and oregano, making sure to season the second layer, then roast in the oven for 30 minutes, or until golden brown and bubbling. A few minutes before it is ready, sprinkle over the grated Parmesan and return to the oven to finish cooking.

NON-FAST DAY: Increase or double the portion size and/or serve with a thin slice of sourdough toast or a wholegrain bread roll.

Prawn Curry with Coconut Milk

Per serving: 338kcals, 25g protein, 9g carbs

I keep frozen foods, such as prawns and edamame beans, in the freezer for healthy last-minute meals like this creamy curry. Frozen fish and veg retain their nutrients well and are often cheaper than fresh. Serve with Cauli Rice (see page 245) or Cabbage Pappardelle (see page 243).

Serves 4
Prep time: 7–10 minutes
Cook time: 10 minutes

   1 tbsp olive oil
   1 medium onion, peeled and diced
   4 garlic cloves, peeled and finely chopped
   2.5cm piece of fresh root ginger, peeled and diced
      (or ½ tsp ground ginger)
   1 tsp paprika
   1 tsp garam masala
   ½ tsp dried chilli flakes (optional)
   1 × 400ml can coconut milk
   100g frozen edamame beans
   500g large frozen cooked prawns, defrosted

1. Place the oil in a large pan with a well-fitting lid over a medium heat. Add the onions and fry gently for about 3–4 minutes, then stir in the garlic, ginger and spices and cook for a further minute.

2. Pour in the coconut milk, cover with the lid and simmer for about 4 minutes.

3. Add the edamame beans and simmer for 1 minute more.

4. Remove from the heat and stir in the prawns. Leave for a minute or so for them to heat through.

TIP: You can defrost the prawns in the microwave, or simply immerse the bag in a bowl of warm water for about 30–60 minutes. If you are more organised, you could take them out of the freezer the night before and leave them in the fridge.

NON-FAST DAY: Increase or double the portion size and/or serve with 2–3 tablespoons of cooked brown rice or a mixture of wild rice and brown basmati.

Simple Salmon with Fennel, Tomatoes and Lemon

Per serving: 354kcals, 26.5g protein, 5g carbs

Salmon, fennel and lemon are a trio of flavours made for one another and they combine here to make a mouth-watering dish that is high in protein, fibre and vitamins. Serve with half a plate of cooked greens.

Serves 2
Prep time: 5 minutes
Cook time: 35 minutes

> 1 fennel bulb, topped and tailed, halved lengthwise and each half sliced crosswise into half-moons about 0.5cm thick
> 120ml hot stock (made with ½ vegetable stock cube)
> 1 tbsp olive oil
> 2 x 120g salmon fillets
> 250g cherry vine tomatoes
> Juice of ½ lemon
> Pinch of dried chilli flakes (optional)

1. Preheat the oven to 200°C/fan 180°C/gas 6.

2. Place the fennel in a medium baking dish and season with salt and freshly ground black pepper. Pour over the hot stock and olive oil and roast in the oven for about 20 minutes.

3. Remove the dish from the oven and place the salm-

on on top of the fennel. Scatter the cherry tomatoes around it, drizzle with the lemon juice and
season once more with freshly ground black
pepper. Sprinkle with chilli flakes, if using, and
roast in the oven for 15 minutes, or until the
salmon is cooked through.

NON-FAST DAY: Increase or double the portion size and/
or serve with wholegrain pasta or 2–3 tablespoons of
cooked brown rice.

Sesame-Crusted Chicken Kiev

Per serving: 372kcals, 31g protein, 0.5g carbs

Using Boursin, a soft cream cheese with herbs and garlic, to stuff the chicken speeds up prep and you still get that luxurious burst of flavour when you cut into the chicken. We have kept this dish keto by avoiding starchy breadcrumbs and crusting it with sesame seeds instead.

Serves 2
Prep time: 5–6 minutes
Cook time: 30 minutes

2 skinless, boneless chicken thighs
3 tbsp sesame seeds
2 tbsp garlic Boursin
1½ tbsp olive oil
½ lemon, sliced in half

1. Preheat the oven to 200°C/fan 180°C/gas 6 and line a baking sheet with non-stick baking paper.

2. Place the chicken thighs between two pieces of non-stick baking paper and bash with a rolling pin until they are half the thickness.

3. Divide the Boursin between the chicken thighs, spreading it over one half of each piece. Season with salt and freshly ground black pepper, then fold the chicken in half to cover the Boursin and press the edges to seal.

4. Tip the sesame seeds onto a plate and dip each thigh into them, ensuring both sides are coated.

5. Place the oil in a non-stick frying pan over a medium heat. When hot, add the chicken and fry for 2 minutes on each side, or until golden. Transfer the thighs to the prepared baking sheet and roast in the oven for 25 minutes.

6. Garnish with a lemon wedge and serve with steamed veg or a mixed salad.

   NON-FAST DAY: Roast small cubes of butternut squash alongside the chicken or serve it with 2–3 tablespoons of cooked wild rice and brown basmati.

Tuscan Lamb Stew with White Beans

Per serving: 355kcals, 26g protein, 17g carbs

An irresistible, melt-in-the-mouth, slow-cooked stew, fragrant with rosemary and garlic and finished with delicious cannellini beans.

Serves 4
Prep time: 10 minutes
Cook time: 1 hour 45 minutes

> 1½ tbsp olive oil
> 400g lamb neck fillet, cut into 3cm cubes
> 1 medium onion, peeled and diced
> 3 garlic cloves, peeled and roughly chopped
> 2 celery sticks, diced
> 1 × 400g can chopped tomatoes
> 1 chicken stock cube
> 3 sprigs of rosemary, leaves picked
> 1 × 400g can cannellini beans, drained

1. Place a medium casserole with a lid over a high heat and add 1 tablespoon of the olive oil. Carefully place the meat in the casserole, without overcrowding it, and fry for about 5 minutes, or until it is nicely browned all over. Remove from the pan and set aside.

2. Add the onion, garlic, celery and the remaining oil (if needed) and fry over a medium heat for 3–4 minutes, stirring often, until softened.

3. Return the meat to the pan, along with the tomatoes, stock cube, rosemary and 250ml water. Bring to the boil, cover with a lid, reduce the heat and simmer for 1½ hours, checking occasionally to make sure it isn't drying out.

4. Add the beans and cook for a final 5 minutes to heat them through. Add extra water to loosen, if needed. Season with salt and freshly ground black pepper.

TIPS: Stirring ½ tablespoon of cider vinegar through just before serving gives a lovely zing to the dish and really brings the flavours to life. You can double the quantities and freeze portions to look forward to at a later date.

NON-FAST DAY: Add an extra can of beans to the stew and/or serve it with 2–3 tablespoons of cooked brown rice.

Wok-Steamed Sea Bass with Pak Choi

Per serving: 233kcals, 20g protein, 4.5g carbs

This dish has a sense of reveal as you lift the lid, releasing a burst of exotic aromas and, as you move the greens, exposing the fish in a puff of steam.

Serves 2
Prep time: 5–7 minutes
Cook time: 10 minutes

> 1 tbsp olive or rapeseed oil
> Dash of sesame oil (optional)
> 2.5cm piece of fresh root ginger, peeled and diced
> 2 fillets of sea bass or another white fish (around 180g combined weight)
> 1–2 spring onions, trimmed and diced
> 2 pak choi, quartered lengthwise
> ½ tsp dried chilli flakes (optional)
> 1 tbsp soy/tamari sauce or Thai fish sauce

1. Place a wok or large frying pan over a medium heat. Add the oils and fry the ginger for 30 seconds.

2. Place the fish and spring onions in the pan, then cover with the pak choi.

3. Sprinkle with the chilli, if using, and drizzle the soy or fish sauce over the top, along with a tablespoon of water. Cover with a lid and cook for 8–10 minutes.

4. Remove from the heat, uncover and push the pak

choi to one side to reveal the fish underneath.

TIPS: If the fillets are thin, they might cook more quickly. Check they are ready by inserting a fork into the middle and pulling it apart slightly – if it is opaque and flaky, it is done; if not, cook for a little longer. If you don't have a lid for your pan or wok, cover it with some foil.

NON-FAST DAY: Serve with wholegrain noodles or 2–3 tablespoons of cooked brown rice.

Tandoori Chicken Kebabs

Per serving: 322kcals, 41g protein, 16g carbs

Brilliant grab-and-go food that tastes equally good hot or cold. Serve with Raita (see page 251) and a generous mixed green salad dressed with a little olive oil and lemon juice.

Serves 2 / makes 4 kebabs
Prep time: 15–20 minutes
Cook time: 25 minutes

- 2 chicken breasts, cut into 2cm cubes
- 2 tbsp full-fat Greek yoghurt
- 1 tbsp tandoori curry powder (or curry powder of choice)
- 4 wooden skewers
- 2 small red onions, peeled and cut into quarters
- 1 medium-large courgette, trimmed and sliced into 1cm rounds
- 1 red or yellow pepper, deseeded and cut into 16 chunks
- 1 tbsp olive oil, to drizzle

1. Preheat the oven to 200°C/fan 180°C/gas 6 and line a baking sheet with non-stick baking paper.

2. Place the chicken, yoghurt and tandoori powder in a bowl, season with salt and freshly ground black pepper and mix well. If time permits, marinate for 30 minutes.

3. Thread a piece of chicken onto a skewer, followed by pieces of onion, courgette and pepper. Repeat the process until all the chicken and veg have been used up and you have four tightly packed skewers.

4. Place the skewers on the prepared baking sheet, drizzle with the olive oil and roast in the oven for 25 minutes.

NON-FAST DAY: Serve with 2–3 tablespoons of cooked brown rice or a wholemeal chapati.

VEG SIDES
(no calorie counting required)

Baked Courgettes with Parmesan

Baking courgettes in this way really enhances their flavour and makes them a versatile side that will complement almost any savoury dish. They are surprisingly filling and work well as a light snack, too.

Serves 2
Prep time: 3–4 minutes
Cook time: 15 minutes

- 2 medium courgettes, trimmed and halved lengthwise
- 1 tbsp olive oil
- 20g Parmesan, finely grated

1. Preheat the oven to 200°C/fan 180°C/gas 6 and line a baking sheet with non-stick baking paper.

2. Place the courgettes cut side up on the prepared baking sheet and drizzle the olive oil all over. Toss to coat thoroughly.

3. Sprinkle the Parmesan over the top, season with freshly ground black pepper and bake in the oven for 15 minutes.

TIP: Scatter 1 tablespoon of capers over just before cooking for added flavour.

Cabbage Pappardelle

An ideal keto alternative to starchy pappardelle pasta.

Serves 2
Prep time: 2 minutes
Cook time: 2 minutes

> 1 sweetheart cabbage (white or savoy works, too), finely shredded
> 1 tbsp olive oil

1. Bring a large pan of salted water to the boil.

2. Gently add the shredded cabbage, bring back to the boil and simmer for 1 minute.

3. Drain, toss with the olive oil, season with salt and freshly ground black pepper and serve.

Creamy Cooked Kale

A side dish of greens that keeps you feeling full for longer. Kale is rich in nutrients and adding fat to it with this creamy, garlicky sauce will help your body absorb them more easily.

Serves 2
Prep time: 1–2 minutes
Cook time: 4 minutes

- 200g curly kale, tough stalks removed and leaves sliced
- 1 tbsp olive oil
- 1 garlic clove, peeled and finely chopped
- 3 tbsp full-fat Greek yoghurt

1. Place the kale and olive oil in a large pan, cover with a lid and cook gently for 2–3 minutes, stirring once or twice.

2. Remove the lid, add the garlic and cook for 1 minute more.

3. Remove from the heat and leave to cool a little before adding the yoghurt. Season with salt and freshly ground black pepper to serve.

TIP: For extra flavour and a bit of crunch, scatter 1 tablespoon of toasted flaked almonds over the top before serving (add 40kcals).

Cauli rice

A great swap for high-carb rice. You can stir in some chopped parsley or coriander, or squeeze over some fresh lemon juice for added flavour.

Serves 2
Prep time: 2 minutes
Cook time: 3–4 minutes

  200g cauliflower, leaves removed

1. Hold the cauliflower at the stalk end and coarsely grate in short, sharp movements in a downward direction to create tiny shavings of cauliflower resembling grains of rice. You can also do this in a food processor but don't let the pieces get too small or they will turn to a paste.

2. Either add the raw cauli rice to a stir-fry, or steam or sauté for 3–4 minutes. You can steam it in a microwave – place in a microwave-proof bowl and cook on high for 2–3 minutes. The rice should retain a bit of bite, like al dente pasta.

Cauliflower Mash

This creamy 'mash' is made with cauliflower instead of potato so is low carb but still tastes great. We add a drizzle of olive oil or a knob of butter to make it even more luscious.

Serves 2
Prep time: 1 minute
Cook time: 15–20 minutes

>   350g cauliflower, broken into small florets
>   ½ tbsp olive oil or a small knob of butter

1. Half fill a saucepan with water and bring to the boil. Add the cauliflower and return to the boil. Cook for 15–20 minutes or until soft.

2. Drain the cauliflower, then return to the pan. Add the olive oil or butter, a couple of pinches of sea salt and lots of freshly ground black pepper and blitz with a stick blender until smooth. You could also leave it to cool slightly and blend it in a food processor.

TIP: You can mash the cauliflower by hand, but it won't be as smooth.

Quick Pickled Red Onion and Radishes

Easy to make and so low in calories, they don't need counting. Pile this on top of fish or use it to add a bit of instant zing to your veg or salad.

Serves 2
Prep time: 10 minutes

> ¼ red onion, peeled and very finely sliced
> 8 radishes, trimmed and very finely sliced
> 1 tbsp live organic cider vinegar

1. Place the red onion and radishes in a bowl, rub in a generous pinch of fine sea salt and set aside for 10 minutes.

2. Mix in the cider vinegar and, if you have time, leave to marinate for up to 30 minutes for the best flavour.

3. Drain off the liquid before eating.

TIP: This pickle can be kept in the fridge for up to 24 hours.

'Pickled' Cucumber

This is actually a ferment, rather than a pickle (which would be sterilised and preserved in vinegar). Fermented foods support your gut microbiome to keep you healthy. Once you get a taste for them, you'll find you are eating them on a daily basis – on scrambled eggs, in salads, with fish, alongside stews and in packed lunches.

> 250ml filtered or spring water
> 1 tbsp sea salt, such as Maldon or kosher salt
> 1 tsp black peppercorns
> 3 sprigs of fresh dill (or 2 tsp dried)
> ½ tsp chilli flakes (optional)
> 1 tsp coriander seeds (optional)
> 1 tsp mustard seeds (optional)
> 2 bay leaves (optional)
> 2 organic, short, knobbly cucumbers, or 1 small–medium regular cucumber (about 400g)

1. You will need a clean (but not sterilised) 1 litre jar with a well-fitting lid.

2. To make a brine, place the filtered water in a mug or bowl and stir in the salt until it has dissolved. Place the peppercorns, dill and your chosen herbs or spices in the jar – any combination should work.

3. Rinse the cucumbers under the tap. Cut them in half lengthwise. Remove the seeds with a spoon. Cut each half in half again lengthwise. Slice the

pieces into sticks that will fit, standing upright, just below the neck of the jar. Try to keep them the same length.

4. Pour over the brine to just cover, then firmly close the lid. (Reserve the remaining brine to top up the level as you eat the cucumbers.) Place the jar in the kitchen at room temperature and out of direct sun.

5. Over the next few days, release the tiny bubbles produced by the ferment. Use a wooden or stainless-steel spoon to press gently on the cucumber and shake it a little from side to side. You will need to 'burp' it once or twice a day for 7–10 days. It is an anaerobic process in which the veg is kept away from air in order to allow it to ferment. The bubbling usually slows after 3–5 days.

6. I like to eat it after 5–7 days, before the flavour gets too strong, but it depends on the surrounding temperature. It should smell sweet and yeasty with a hint of cucumber. You can test it by cutting a piece off with a clean knife. When it is ready, place the jar in the fridge and the fermentation will almost stop. If it has brown spots, smells bad or goes mushy, then discard it. It will keep for a few months in the fridge.

TIP: Filtered water doesn't contain chlorine, which can reduce fermentation.

Dressings

You can use one of these dressings to pep up your salad or veg as an add-on without having to count the calories, as they are all less than 100 cals per serving.

Olive Oil and Mustard

Serves 2

2 tbsp olive oil
1 tbsp live apple cider vinegar
1 tsp Dijon mustard

1. Place all the ingredients in a jar and shake until emulsified. Season with salt and freshly ground black pepper to taste.

   TIP: To get ahead, make double or triple the recipe and keep it in the fridge for when needed.

Yoghurt and Lemon

Serves 2

4 tbsp full-fat Greek yoghurt
2 tbsp good-quality full-fat mayonnaise
Zest and juice of 1 lemon

1. Mix all the ingredients together in a small bowl or jug. Season with salt and freshly ground black pepper to taste.

Raita

Serves 2

4 tbsp full-fat Greek yoghurt
¼ cucumber, grated
Pinch of cumin seeds

1. Mix all the ingredients together in a small bowl or jug. Season with salt and freshly ground black pepper to taste.

OCCASIONAL TREATS

High-Protein Seeded Bread Rolls

Per serving: 224kcals, 9g protein, 11g carbs

This is adapted from a classic keto bread recipe. It may not taste quite like your usual bread but it is remarkably low in carbs and high in nutrients, protein and fibre.

Makes 6
Prep time: 15 minutes
Cook time: 35–40 minutes

> 140g ground almonds
> 60g psyllium husk
> 2 tsp baking powder
> 2 tbsp mixed seeds (any of the following or a mixture: sunflower, pumpkin, sesame, poppy, flax)
> 1 tsp sea salt
> 3 egg whites
> 250ml warm water
> 2 tsp cider vinegar

1. Preheat the oven to 180°C/fan 160°C/gas 4 and line a baking sheet with non-stick baking paper.

2. Mix all the dry ingredients together in a large bowl.

3. Add the egg whites, warm water and cider vinegar

and give it all a quick mix until well combined. The mixture should form a dough-like ball.

4. With a few drops of olive oil on your hands to prevent sticking, shape the dough into 6 rolls and place on the prepared baking sheet. Bake in the oven for 35–40 minutes, or until the base sounds hollow when tapped. And if, rather than rolls, you want more of a sandwich pocket, shape the dough into flatter, squarer pieces and remove them sooner from the oven.

Dark Choc Bites

Per serving: 41kcals, 1.5g protein, 4.5g carbs

These scrumptious bites will not only satisfy your cravings for a sweet but also deliver a burst of protein and fibre.

Makes 12
Prep time: 5–7 minutes
Cook time: 15 minutes

> 1 ripe banana, peeled and mashed
> 6 tbsp ground almonds
> 4–6 dried pitted dates, diced
> 2 tbsp unsweetened cocoa powder
> 1 tsp vanilla extract
> ½ tbsp coconut oil

1. Preheat the oven to 200°C/fan 180°C/gas 6 and line a baking sheet with non-stick baking paper.

2. Place all the ingredients in a small bowl and mix with a fork until combined.

3. Use a teaspoon to spoon 12 small balls of the mixture onto the prepared baking sheet. Flatten each one slightly with a fork and bake for about 15 minutes.

Raspberry Fool

Per serving: 107kcals, 4g protein, 6g carbs

This elegant raspberry dessert is deceptively easy to make and won't spike blood sugars.

Serves 2
Prep time: 5 minutes

  140g full-fat Greek yoghurt
  ½ tsp vanilla extract
  ½ tsp honey
  50g frozen raspberries, defrosted

1. Mix the yoghurt, vanilla and honey together in a bowl.

2. Divide the yoghurt mixture and raspberries between two small bowls. Gently stir the raspberries through the yoghurt, creating a marbled effect, to serve.

TIPS: Add 10g grated chocolate (70% cocoa solids) for added decadence. Frozen raspberries are slightly better than fresh here, as they release lots of lovely juice when they defrost. If you're using fresh, simply mash with the back of a fork before adding to the yoghurt.

Strawberries Dipped in Dark Chocolate and Chopped Pistachios

Per serving: 184kcals, 4g protein, 18g carbs

A classic chocolate treat which is also keto-friendly. Strawberries are sweet but surprisingly low in sugar, while dark chocolate has anti-inflammatory properties and may reduce heart disease. Enjoy!

Serves 2
Prep time: 10 minutes

> 14 strawberries, washed and dried, leafy tops left on
> 30g dark chocolate (70% cocoa solids), melted
> 2 tbsp pistachios, finely chopped

1. Dip each strawberry into the melted chocolate, then into the pistachios.

2. Allow to cool and harden before serving.

TIP: Add a pinch of dried chilli flakes or freshly ground black pepper to the pistachios for a touch of heat.

ADD-ONS

Protein

Maintaining an adequate protein intake is important when you are fasting. During Stage 1, we recommend you eat at least 50g daily. Then, as you transition to normal eating, you should ramp your intake up – see page 59. By Stage 3, the recommended amounts are 70–80g per day for women, and 90–100g for men.

Here are some examples of how to top up your protein on days when you are a bit low on it – even if your calories then increase to closer to 1000. (NB. If you are vegan, you will find you need to top up your protein every day and will go over 1000 calories on most days, unless you are using a protein powder – see page 118. Don't worry too much about this, as you will still be losing weight, and it's not *all* about the calories!)

Meat

- **1 tbsp (about 7g) chopped dry-fried bacon** (23kcals/1.7g protein) – scatter over the Lunchbox Salad
- **1 tbsp (10g) diced chorizo** (40kcals/2.7g protein) – sprinkle on the Pea and Mint Soup
- **75g cooked chicken breast** (115kcals/22.6g protein) – serve alongside the Goat's Cheese Frittata

Fish

45g drained tuna in oil (85kcals/5g protein) – add to the Roasted Broccoli and Kale

4 drained anchovies in oil (23kcals/3g protein) – add 1 anchovy to each Cheesy Asparagus Prosciutto Bite

75g cooked prawns (59kcals/10g protein) – add to the Prawn Curry with Coconut Milk

Dairy and Egg

1 tbsp (about 40g) full-fat live Greek yoghurt (53kcals/2.2g protein) – dollop on top of the Rapid Bircher

10g Parmesan (42kcals/3.5g protein) – grate and sprinkle over the Baked Meatballs with Mozzarella

15g full-fat feta (37kcals/2.3g protein) – scatter over the Easy Chicken, Spinach and Tomato Casserole

30g Cheddar, about matchbox sized (124kcals/7.5g protein) – grate and sprinkle over the Spinach and Ham Omelette

30g halloumi, sliced, lightly fried in 1 tsp olive oil for 4–5 mins (145kcals/6g protein) – serve along side the Aubergine Parmigiana

1 medium egg (78kcals/7.7g protein) – have an extra egg with the Microwave Eggs with Spinach and Mackerel

Grains, seeds and nuts

- **15g mixed seeds** (55kcals/2.2g protein) – sprinkle over a green salad and serve alongside the Tandoori Chicken Kebabs
- **2 tsp (about 10g) sesame seeds** (60kcals/2.1g protein) – sprinkle over the Quick Veg and Salmon Stir-Fry with Ginger and Oyster Sauce
- **80g cooked shelled edamame beans** (110kcals/9g protein) – serve alongside the Baked White Fish with Parmesan Crust
- **15g almonds** (95kcals/3.8g protein) – roughly chop and toast in a dry frying pan, then sprinkle on top of the Tuscan Lamb Stew
- **Handful of nuts**, around 30g, e.g. walnuts or hazel nuts (185kcals/7.6g protein) – toast in a dry frying pan and sprinkle over Keto Pancakes
- **100g cooked Puy lentils** (143kcals/10.6g protein) – stir into the Simple Saag or serve alongside the Sesame-Crusted Chicken Kiev
- **100g canned beans** (109cals/7g protein)
- **100g cooked quinoa** (185cals/6g protein)
- **100g tofu** (123cals/12.5g protein)

Simple Greens and Non-Starchy Veg

Greens and non-starchy vegetables are such an important part of your diet that you should eat them freely without counting the calories. Examples of greens and non-starchy veg include: cabbage, spring greens, chard, kale, pak choi, cavolo nero, spinach, green beans, mange tout, courgettes, broccoli, tomatoes and salad leaves.

Adding flavour will help you eat these veggies regularly. Try first just adding some seasoning – flaked sea salt or soy sauce and freshly ground pepper will make a big difference for a start. A pinch of dried chilli flakes, for lovers of heat, or a little crushed garlic are also good, and a squeeze of lemon or lime juice over some broccoli or cabbage goes really well.

For salad dressings, see pages 250–51. And here are some other low-calorie ways to add flavour:

- **1 tsp butter** (25kcals) – good on any veg
- **1 tsp olive oil** (27kcals) – good on any veg
- **1 tsp hoisin sauce** (12kcals) – try this on wilted spinach or steamed broccoli florets
- **1 tsp nigella seeds** (32kcals) – sprinkle over green beans or cabbage
- **1 tsp grated Parmesan** (8kcals) – scatter on top of roasted courgettes or cauliflower florets

TIP: Remember, if you want to add a little something to your plate, *always* choose a protein add-on or some non-starchy veg, rather than carbohydrates.

Meal planner – 3 meals a day

Day	
1	Keto Pancakes with Yoghurt and Berries (p166) Cheesy Asparagus Prosciutto Bites (p193) Steamed Fish with Tomato and Pepper Sauce (p208) Raspberry Fool (p255)
2	Rapid Bircher with Apple and Cinnamon (p168) Pea and Mint Soup with 15g feta add-on (p177) Pulled Pork with Cider Vinegar (p262)
3	Scrambled Eggs with Smoked Salmon, Feta and Avocado with 15g mixed seeds add-on (p169) Goat's Cheese Frittata with Greens and Diced Figs (p183) Black Bean Chilli with Cabbage Pappardelle (p218 and p243)
4	Spinach and Ham Omelette (p187) Curried Smoked Haddock Chowder (p181) Speedy One-Pan Thai Red Curry with Salmon (p222)
5	Cheese and Chive Muffins (p173) Protein Wrap with Smoked Salmon, Cream Cheese and Capers (p185) Aubergine Parmigiana with Lentils (p228)
6	Cashew, Vanilla and Fig Breakfast Shake (p176) Waldorf Salad (p191) Black Bean Chilli (p218) Two Dark Choc Bites (p254)
7	Microwave Eggs with Spinach and Mackerel (p175) Chunky Courgette and Dill Soup with Prawns (p179) Cauliflower Rice Risotto with Chicken, Edamame and Roasted Red Peppers (p214)

	Total cals	carbs	protein
	844	40.8g	49g
	885	33g	51g
	848	28g	50.2g
	830	17g	73.5g
	895	19.5g	53g
	854	44g	53g
	816	17g	62g

Extra days – 3 meals

Day	
1	Rapid Bircher with Apple and Cinnamon (p168)
	Quick Veg and Salmon Stir-Fry with Ginger and Oyster Sauce with 2 tsp sesame seeds add-on (p226)
	Wok-Steamed Sea Bass with Pak Choi (p238)
2	Keto Pancakes with Yoghurt and Berries (p166)
	Pea and Mint Soup (p177)
	Sesame-Crusted Chicken Kiev (p234)
	Strawberries Dipped in Dark Chocolate and Chopped Pistachios (p256)

Sample vegetarian days – 3 meals

Day	
1	Keto Pancakes with Yoghurt and Berries (p166)
	Goat's Cheese Frittata with Greens and Diced Figs (p183)
	Simple Saag with Tandoori Halloumi (p201)
2	Cashew, Vanilla and Fig Breakfast Shake (p176)
	Protein Wrap with Beetroot, Rocket & Feta (p185)
	Roasted Broccoli and Kale with Halloumi and Harissa with 15g mixed seeds add-on (p199)
3	Cheese and Chive Muffins x 2 (p173)
	Lunchbox Salad of Broccoli, Feta and Piquanté Peppers with 15g mixed seeds add-on (p194)
	Aubergine Parmigiana with Lentils (p228)

	Total cals	carbs	protein
	948	29.5g	51.1g
	904	32g	51g

	Total cals	carbs	protein
	1004	34.5g	53g
	913	31.5g	51.2g
	1085	24g	50.2g

Meal planner – 2 meals a day

Day	
1	Tandoori Chicken Kebabs with Raita (p240 and 251) Tuscan Lamb Stew with White Beans (p236) Two Dark Choc Bites (p254)
2	Easy Chicken, Spinach and Tomato Soup (p211) Prawn Curry with Coconut Milk with 80g edamame beans add-on (p230)
3	Breakfast Traybake (p164) Protein Salad with Tuna, Roasted Red Peppers, Edamame and Harissa (p189)
4	Microwave Eggs with Spinach and Mackerel (p175) Steamed Fish with Tomato and Pepper Sauce (p208) Raspberry Fool (p255)
5	Protein Salad with Tuna, Roasted Red Peppers, Edamame and Harissa (p189) Speedy One-Pan Thai Red Curry with Salmon (p222)
6	Simple Saag with Tandoori Halloumi (p201) Pulled Pork with Cider Vinegar (p220)
7	Scrambled Eggs with Smoked Salmon, Feta and Avocado (p169) Curried Smoked Haddock Chowder (p181) Strawberries Dipped in Dark Chocolate (p256)

	Total cals	carbs	protein
	811	42g	72.2g
	841	37.5g	58.5g
	797	16g	52g
	840	36g	52g
	837	18.5g	53g
	903	28g	56.7g
	785	30g	57.5g

Extra days – 2 meals

Day	
1	Lunchbox Salad of Broccoli, Feta and Piquanté Peppers with 1 medium hard-boiled egg add-on (p194) Beef Stroganoff (p216) Two Dark Choc Bites (p254)
2	Protein Wrap with Smoked Salmon, Cream Cheese and Capers (p185) Steamed Fish with Tomato and Pepper Sauce (p208)

Sample vegetarian days – 2 meals

Day	
1	Goat's Cheese Frittata with Greens and Diced Figs (p183) Simple Saag with Tandoori Halloumi (p201) Strawberries Dipped in Dark Chocolate and Chopped Pistachios (p256)
2	Roasted Broccoli and Kale with Halloumi and Harissa with 80g edamame beans add-on (p199) Aubergine Parmigiana with Lentils with a High-Protein Seeded Bread Roll (p228 and 252)

	Total cals	carbs	protein
	973	23.5g	51.7g
	813	27.5g	57g

	Total cals	carbs	protein
	1001	48g	49g
	1052	30.5g	50g

Endnotes

1 Obesity and overweight factsheet, World Health Organization. www.who.int/news-room/fact-sheets/detail/obesity-and-overweight &

Obesity Update, OECD, www.oecd.org/els/health-systems/Obesity-Update-2017.pdf

2 Article, *Washington Post*. www.washingtonpost.com/news/wonk/wp/2016/01/29/the-age-when-you-gain-the-most-weight/

3 Do weight perceptions among obese adults in Great Britain match clinical definitions? *BMJ* Open. https://bmjopen.bmj.com/content/4/11/e005561.full?sid=ef1e9018-cd8a-4c5e-8ed9-f52b04290546

4 Covid-19 and metabolic syndrome: could diet be the key? Dr Marianne Demasi. https://ebm.bmj.com/content/26/1/1

5 Prevalence of Overweight, Obesity, and Severe Obesity Among Adults Aged 20 and Over: United States, 1960–1962 Through 2015–2016, Centres for Disease Control and Prevention. www.cdc.gov/nchs/data/hestat/obesity_adult_15_16/obesity_adult_15_16.htm

6 Effects of n-3 Polyunsaturated Fatty Acid Supplementation in the Prevention and Treatment of Depressive Disorders—A Systematic Review and Meta-Analysis, *Nutrients*, 2021. www.ncbi.nlm.nih.gov/pmc/articles/PMC8064470/

7 Regular fish consumption and age-related brain gray matter loss, *Am. J. Prev. Med.*, 2014. https://pubmed.ncbi.nlm.nih.gov/25084680/

8 Quantifying greenhouse gas emissions from global aquaculture, *Scientific Reports*, 2020. www.nature.com/articles/s41598-020-68231-8

9 Egg consumption and risk of cardiovascular disease: three large prospective US cohort studies, systematic review, and updated meta-analysis. *BMJ*, 2020. www.bmj.com/content/368/bmj.m513

10 Primary Prevention of Cardiovascular Disease with a Mediterranean Diet Supplemented with Extra-Virgin Olive Oil or Nuts. *The New England Journal of Medicine*, 2018. www.nejm.org/doi/full/10.1056/nejmoa1800389

11 Nutrition and health: The issue is not food, nor nutrients, so much as processing, Cambridge University Press, 2009. https://doi.org/10.1017/S1368980009005291

12 NOVA. The star shines bright. *World Nutrition*, 2016. https://worldnutritionjournal.org/index.php/wn/article/view/5

13 The Coca-Cola Company, PepsiCo and Nestlé named top plastic polluters for the third year in a row. www.breakfreefromplastic.org/2020/12/02/top-plastic-polluters-of-2020/

14 The Global Commitment: Progress Report. https://ellenmacarthurfoundation.org/global-commitment/signatory-reports

15 The UN Decade of Nutrition, the NOVA food classification and the trouble with ultra-processing. Cambridge University Press, 2017. www.cambridge.org/core/journals/public-health-nutrition/article/un-decade-of-nutrition-the-nova-food-classification-and-the-trouble-with-ultraprocessing/2A9776922A28F8F757BDA32C3266AC2A

16 Development and validation of a food frequency questionnaire in Spain. *Int. J. Epidemiol.*, 1993. https://pubmed.ncbi.nlm.nih.gov/8359969/

17 Trends in Consumption of Ultraprocessed Foods Among US Youths Aged 2-19 Years, 1999-2018. *JAMA*, 2021. https://jamanetwork.com/journals/jama/article-abstract/2782866

18 Ultra-Processed Diets Cause Excess Calorie Intake and Weight Gain: An Inpatient Randomized Controlled Trial of Ad Libitum

Food Intake. *Cell Metab.*, 2019. https://pubmed.ncbi.nlm.nih.gov/31105044/

19 How to eat like the animals for good health, 2020. www.sydney.edu.au/news-opinion/news/2020/05/06/How-to-eat-like-the-animals-for-good-health.html

20 Testing protein leverage in lean humans: a randomised controlled experimental study. *PLoS One*, 2011. https://pubmed.ncbi.nlm.nih.gov/22022472/

21 The Potential Role of Protein Leverage in the US Obesity Epidemic. *Obesity* (Silver Spring), 2019. https://pubmed.ncbi.nlm.nih.gov/31095898/

22 What's on your table? How America's diet has changed over the decades. Pew Research Center, 2016. https://www.pewresearch.org/fact-tank/2016/12/13/whats-on-your-table-how-americas-diet-has-changed-over-the-decades/

23 Low-Protein Intakes and Poor Diet Quality Associate with Functional Limitations in US Adults with Diabetes: A 2005–2016 NHANES Analysis. *Nutrients*, 2021. www.mdpi.com/2072-6643/13/8/2582

24 Introduction to Protein Summit 2.0: continued exploration of the impact of high-quality protein on optimal health. *Amer. J. Clin. Nutr.*, 2015. https://academic.oup.com/ajcn/article/101/6/1317S/4564491

25 Benefits and safety of dietary protein for bone health – an expert consensus paper endorsed by the European Society for Clinical and Economical Aspects of Osteoporosis, Osteoarthritis, and Musculoskeletal Diseases and by the International Osteoporosis Foundation. *Osteoporosis Int.*, 2018. https://pubmed.ncbi.nlm.nih.gov/29740667/

26 Protein Intake and Functional Integrity in Aging: The Framingham Heart Study Offspring. *The Journals of Gerontology*, 2020. https://academic.oup.com/biomedgerontology/

article/75/1/123/5106141

27 Protein and Amino Acid Requirements during Pregnancy. *Adv. Nutr.*, 2016. www.ncbi.nlm.nih.gov/pmc/articles/PMC4942872/

28 Protein Requirements and Recommendations for Older People: A Review. *Nutrients*, 2015. https://www.ncbi.nlm.nih.gov/pmc/articles/PMC4555150/

29 Four grams of glucose. *Am. J. Physiol. Endocrinol. Metab.*, 2009. www.ncbi.nlm.nih.gov/pmc/articles/PMC2636990/

30 Efficacy and safety of very low calorie ketogenic diet (VLCKD) in patients with overweight and obesity: A systematic review and meta-analysis. *Rev. Endocr. Metab. Disord.*, 2020. https://pubmed.ncbi.nlm.nih.gov/31705259/

31 Obesity treatment by very low-calorie-ketogenic diet at two years: reduction in visceral fat and on the burden of disease. *Endocrine*, 2016. https://pubmed.ncbi.nlm.nih.gov/27623967/

32 The Starvation Experiment. https://eatingdisorders.dukehealth.org/education/resources/starvation-experiment

33 Persistent metabolic adaptation 6 years after "The Biggest Loser" competition. *Obesity (Silver Spring)*, 2016. https://pubmed.ncbi.nlm.nih.gov/27136388/

34 Energy compensation and adiposity in humans. *Current Biology*, 2021. www.cell.com/current-biology/fulltext/S0960-9822(21)01120-9

35 Changes in breakfast and dinner timings can reduce body fat, 2018. www.surrey.ac.uk/news/changes-breakfast-and-dinner-timings-can-reduce-body-fat

36 Ten-Hour Time-Restricted Eating Reduces Weight, Blood Pressure, and Atherogenic Lipids in Patients with Metabolic Syndrome. *Cell Metabolism*, 2019. https://www.cell.com/cell-metabolism/fulltext/S1550-4131(19)30611-4?_returnURL=https%3A%2F%2Flinkinghub.elsevier.com%2Fretrieve%2

Fpii%2FS1550413119306114%3Fshowall%3Dtrue

37 Effects of Intermittent Fasting on Health, Aging, and Disease. *New Eng. J. Med.*, 2019. www.nejm.org/doi/full/10.1056/nejmra1905136

38 Effects of Ketogenic Dieting on Body Composition, Strength, Power, and Hormonal Profiles in Resistance Training Men. *J. Strength Cond. Res.*, 2020. https://pubmed.ncbi.nlm.nih.gov/28399015/

39 Long-term weight-loss maintenance: a meta-analysis of US studies. *Am. J. Clin. Nutr.*, 2001. https://pubmed.ncbi.nlm.nih.gov/11684524/

40 Reversing Type 2 Diabetes and ongoing remission. www.ncl.ac.uk/magres/research/diabetes/reversal/#publicinformation

41 Ethnic Differences in BMI and Disease Risk, *Obesity Prevention Source*. https://www.hsph.harvard.edu/obesity-prevention-source/ethnic-differences-in-bmi-and-disease-risk/

42 Blood Pressure and Stroke: An Overview of Published Reviews. www.ahajournals.org/doi/10.1161/01.str.0000116869.64771.5a

43 Adapted from 'Primary prevention of cardiovascular disease with a Mediterranean Diet, *New Eng. J. Med.*, 2013.

44 A randomised controlled trial of dietary improvement for adults with major depression (the 'SMILES' trial). *BMC*, 2017. https://bmcmedicine.biomedcentral.com/articles/10.1186/s12916-017-0791-y

45 Durability of a primary care-led weight-management intervention for remission of type 2 diabetes: 2-year results of the DiRECT open-label, cluster-randomised trial. *Diabetes & Endocrin.*, 2019. www.thelancet.com/journals/landia/article/PIIS2213-8587(19)30068-3/fulltext

46 Joint association between accelerometry-measured daily combination of time spent in physical activity, sedentary behaviour and

sleep and all-cause mortality: a pooled analysis of six prospective cohorts using compositional analysis. *Brit J. Sports Med.*, 2021. bjsports-2020-102345 DOI: 10.1136/bjsports-2020-102345

47 *Med. & Science in Sports and Exercise*, 2021. https://journals.lww.com/acsm-msse/Abstract/2021/01000/Metabolic_Effect_of_Breaking_Up_Prolonged_Sitting.18.aspx

48 Do stair climbing exercise "snacks" improve cardiorespiratory fitness? *Applied Physiology, Nutrition, and Metabolism*, 2019. https://cdnsciencepub.com/doi/10.1139/apnm-2018-0675

49 Health effects of dietary risks in 195 countries, 1990–2017: a systematic analysis for the Global Burden of Disease Study 2017. *Lancet*, 2019. www.thelancet.com/article/S0140-6736(19)30041-8/fulltext

50 Assessing the healthiness of UK food companies' product portfolios using food sales and nutrient composition data. *PLoS One*, 2021. https://journals.plos.org/plosone/article?id=10.1371/journal.pone.0254833

Before and after measurements

	Weight	Waist	Blood pressure
Week 1			
Week 2			
Week 3			
Week 4			
Week 5			
Week 6			

	Weight	Waist	Blood pressure
Week 7			
Week 8			
Week 9			
Week 10			
Week 11			
Week 12			

Notes

Notes

Index

Dr Michael Mosley is a science presenter, journalist and executive producer. After training to be a doctor at the Royal Free Hospital in London, he spent 30 years at the BBC, where he made numerous science documentaries. Now freelance, he is the author of several bestselling books, *The Fast Diet*, *The 8-Week Blood Sugar Diet*, *The Clever Guts Diet* and *The Fast 800*. He is married with four children.

Dr Clare Bailey, wife of Michael Mosley, is a GP of 30 years who has supported hundreds of patients to lose weight, reduce their blood sugars and put their diabetes into remission at her surgery in Buckinghamshire. A health writer and journalist with a particular interest in parenting and childhood nutrition, she is the author of the bestselling *8-Week Blood Sugar Diet Recipe Book*, *Clever Guts Diet Recipe Book*, *Fast 800 Recipe Book* and *Fast 800 Easy*. Instagram @drclarebailey